# WOMEN,
# FOOD,
# AND
# HORMONES

ALSO BY SARA GOTTFRIED, MD

*The Hormone Cure*

*The Hormone Reset Diet*

*Younger*

*Brain Body Diet*

# WOMEN, FOOD, AND HORMONES

A Four-Week Plan to Achieve
Hormonal Balance, Lose Weight,
and Feel Like Yourself Again

## Sara Gottfried, MD

Houghton Mifflin Harcourt
Boston ▪ New York
2021

For information about permission to reproduce selections
from this book, write to trade.permissions@hmhco.com or to
Permissions, Houghton Mifflin Harcourt Publishing Company,
3 Park Avenue, 19th Floor, New York, New York 10016.

hmhbooks.com

Library of Congress Cataloging-in-Publication Data
Names: Gottfried, Sara, author.
Title: Women, food, and hormones : a 4-week plan to achieve hormonal balance,
lose weight, and feel like yourself again / Sara Gottfried, MD.
Description: Boston : Houghton Mifflin Harcourt, 2021. |
Includes bibliographical references and index.
Identifiers: LCCN 2021004079 (print) | LCCN 2021004080 (ebook) |
ISBN 9780358345411 (hardcover) | ISBN 9780358578437 | ISBN 9780358578840 |
ISBN 9780358346210 (ebook)
Subjects: LCSH: Reducing diets. | Ketogenic diet. | Low-carbohydrate diet. | Menopause —
Popular works. | Middle-aged women — Health and Hygiene — Popular works.
Classification: LCC RM222.2 .G6817 2021 (print) | LCC RM222.2 (ebook) |
DDC 613.2/5—dc23
LC record available at https://lccn.loc.gov/2021004079
LC ebook record available at https://lccn.loc.gov/2021004080

Book design by Chrissy Kurpeski

Printed in the United States of America
1 2021
4500833039

This book presents, among other things, the research and ideas of its author. It is not intended to be a substitute for consultation with a professional health-care practitioner. Consult with your health-care practitioner before starting any diet or other medical regimen. The publisher and the author disclaim responsibility for any adverse effects resulting directly or indirectly from information contained in this book.

Some names and identifying details have been changed.

Carrot Cake Shake recipe adapted from Kelly LeVeque; Tahini Bread, Cauliflower Ceviche, Halibut with Almond Crust recipes courtesy of Nathalie Hadi; Tofu Masala Soup recipe courtesy of Anu French, MD; Shakshuka, Crispy Cucumber Salad with Tahini Dressing, Tahini Dressing; Kimchi, Shirataki, and Bok Choy Bowl; Lemon-Herb Mojo, Slow-Cooker Chicken, Nut-Crusted Chicken Fingers, Almond-Coconut Macaroons, Chocolate-Avocado "Ice Cream," Avocado-Lime Sorbet recipes adapted from *Brain Body Diet* by Sara Gottfried, MD; Egg-Avocado Bake, Mayonnaise, Ranch Dressing, Seaweed Salad, Kale and Caesar Salad, Alkaline Broth with Collagen, Chicken Bone Broth, Beef Bone Broth, Salmon and Avocado Bowl with Miso Dressing, Black Cod with Miso, Braised Turmeric-Cinnamon Chicken, Beef and Vegetable Stew, No-Bake Coconut Love Bites, Dark Chocolate–Coconut Pudding recipes adapted from *Younger* by Sara Gottfried, MD.

# CONTENTS

# PART I

# Understanding Women, Food, and Hormones

# INTRODUCTION:
## The Language of Hormones

Few things on earth are as misunderstood as women, food, and hormones.

I've seen it again and again in my practice: women come to me feeling overtired, cranky, frazzled, and — inevitably — lamenting the extra pounds they've put on despite their best efforts to exercise and eat right. More often than not, these issues start when women enter their midthirties. My patients notice that it's harder to maintain a healthy weight. Those holiday pounds are harder to shave off, even with January's discipline. The diet plans that worked in the past don't seem to work anymore. Even more disheartening, diets that work for male co-workers and partners don't seem to work the same for them.

My patients are often surprised when I explain that the solution to their symptoms can't be found by counting calories or clocking miles on the treadmill, but by learning to speak the language of hormones.

I know what you're thinking: *hormones?* Yes, hormones.

As a board-certified physician who has been practicing medicine for more than twenty-five years, and precision medicine for the past fifteen, I can tell you without a doubt that you cannot achieve true health without achieving hormonal health and balance. I can help you do just that, using science that honors your body.

What does that mean, exactly? When your diet and lifestyle support your hormones, your hormones will support you. It's like a cool breeze on a hot summer day when your food tells your body to burn fat and promote health. You flip a metabolic switch, and your body is transformed. This is particularly welcome after age thirty-five, when the scale gets harder to budge!

What makes the scale stick? Your metabolism is grinding to a halt. Your metabolism is the sum of all of the biochemical reactions in your body, including those related to your hormones, that dictate how you feel and determine how fast or slow you burn calories. Metabolism is the foundation of your health, today and tomorrow. When you learn to speak the language of hormones, you can improve metabolism, lose fat, and finally maintain a healthy body weight by burning rather than storing fat. At the same time, you resolve nagging, unpleasant symptoms like fatigue, cravings, moodiness, insomnia, and a weak immune system. Too many health plans don't work because they are designed by men, for men, and not for women's complex hormonal needs. I'm going to show you how to achieve this ultimate goal in a way that *honors your unique female biology.*

## WHAT TO EAT?

Many of my patients want to know what to eat to stay healthy, but they feel confused. I don't blame them: there's so much conflicting information out there. And over time, the answer has changed. In the 1980s, fat was villainized; later, sugar. As fasting protocols became all the rage, the focus shifted from *what should I eat* to *when should I eat.* Very often my patients come to me having tried these various plans, only to find they just gained weight, or they are so overwhelmed with choices, they stay in the same food rut because they aren't sure which plan is right for them.

What *not* to eat is easy. The truth is, a powerful link exists between consumption of processed food, weight gain, and poor immunity. More than half of Americans' caloric intake now comes from ultraprocessed foods: chips, soda, cookies, candy, and other Frankenfoods. The results are plain to see. Not only did the United States fare worse than many other countries during the COVID-19 pandemic, but also our rates of weight gain, obesity, diabetes, cardiovascular disease, cancer, and depression are high. The food we eat sets us up to be extraordinarily unhealthy, making us vulnerable to chronic disease and to viruses like COVID-19.

My answer to this age-old question of what to eat? *Eat for your hormones.*

Food is the backbone of the hormones you make. When it comes to your health and metabolism, food is medicine. I'm going to clear up the confusion about what's healthy and what's not and give you all the support you need to be successful. I'll share a proven plan that's designed to meet your hormonal needs and help you reclaim your health in four weeks.

To start, consuming healthy fat is especially critical to long-term hormone balance. Healthy fat makes you feel more satisfied, and it slows down or eliminates the spikes in blood sugar that can make you accumulate fat. You need moderate protein — not so much that it turns into sugar, but not so little that your muscles start to break down. Some guidelines you've likely heard about before are important too, such as avoiding sugar and excess refined carbohydrates, enjoying healthy fats like extra-virgin olive oil and avocado oil, and even following fasting protocols. I've integrated these strategies into a single cohesive approach I call the Gottfried Protocol, which will allow you to switch your metabolism from stuck and inflexible to unstuck and flexible. As you do so, you'll lengthen your health span (that is, your healthy life span), support your immune system, and improve your overall health.

## HOW NUTRITION AND I EVOLVED TOGETHER

I didn't learn the answers to these food queries at Harvard Medical School or the University of California at San Francisco, where I served my internship and residency in obstetrics and gynecology. In fact, during my medical education, nutrition and lifestyle approaches to health were tolerated but never championed. Yet this lack of interest was a scientific contradiction that has since been evolving. We now know that better diet and lifestyle are the most important drivers of disease prevention and reversal for the people who are willing to commit to them. Science has documented the evidence for this fact many times over, though the discoveries have been largely ignored by mainstream medicine.

Look no further than the hormone insulin. You've probably heard about it. Insulin's primary job is to move glucose into your cells, thereby lowering the glucose in your blood. It's a key hormone in the treatment and prevention of diabetes. The scientific literature demonstrates that dietary and lifestyle approaches to diabetes — a condition in which cells become numb to the hormone insulin — work better than medications,[1] perhaps because they don't disrupt normal biochemistry and instead help an individual return to a state of homeostasis, or balance. Yet few physicians (myself included) learned how to use nutritional intervention or how to guide changes to behavior and lifestyle.

As a result, I had to teach myself how to do these things. Fortunately, I had an ideal patient, one who struggled with multiple hormone problems: *me*. My personal struggle to balance my hormones has informed my career as a physician and writer. I come to this topic as a doctor and scientist, but also as a case study.

In medical school, I was taught to advise patients to exercise more and eat less if they wanted to lose weight. When I followed that advice, I made my hormone imbalance worse because the essential role of metabolic hormones, and how they function in women, was missing from the equation. In my thirties, I began to battle depression, premenstrual syndrome, and belly fat. I wrestled with my weight because my levels of testosterone, growth hormone, estrogen, and progesterone were too low, and my insulin and cortisol were too high. That made me get stressed about the small stuff. I'd work out for hours with nothing to show for it on the bathroom scale or in my musculature. I was on a mostly vegan diet, and I wasn't getting the healthy fat I needed to synthesize these hormones in my body. Seemingly overnight, my triceps area became flabby. There were longitudinal lines on my nails, and I noticed weird fatty "cushions" at my knees. *What?!* Worst of all, I felt frazzled and overwhelmed much of the time; I lacked inner peace. If you're like me or my patients, you may not notice that your hormones are off kilter. Instead, you may observe difficulty with sleeping, with losing the baby weight, or with low sex drive. Maybe your workouts don't seem to have an impact.

After being offered an antidepressant and the birth control pill to address my afflictions, I just felt they were not the right treatment. Then, with a simple blood test, I discovered my hormones were out of balance. As I corrected my hormones, I learned they were the root cause of my troubles. I began seeing hormone imbalance in nearly all of my patients who were medicated by their well-meaning doctors. I wrote several books about how to balance hormones: *The Hormone Cure, The Hormone Reset Diet, Younger,* and *Brain Body Diet.* However, I didn't fully connect the dots between hormones, food, and metabolic flexibility until now. My goal is to save you time in finding a solution. I uncovered what worked, and what didn't, to get my hormones back in the target zone, burn fat, and lose weight. You can too.

Thankfully, the culture of medicine is changing. Science and technology are advancing. My practice has evolved, thanks to these recent developments.

Today I help my patients personalize the way they eat in order to balance their hormones. I do this through the practice of *precision medicine.* Defined by the National Institutes of Health as an emerging approach to disease treatment and prevention, precision medicine takes into account individual variability in genes, environment, and lifestyle.[2] Its practitioners use every means possible: wearable sensors like watches, rings, and continuous glucose monitors; nutrient trackers, Bluetooth body-composition scales in the bathroom at home, and food log apps; stress tests, stress hormone tests, heart rate variability, and other measures of recovery; genetic and epigenetic panels; home lab testing (yes, including poop tests), finger pricks, and computation to analyze these complex data flows. This is a collaborative process involving the patient and other clinicians; we share a common dashboard documenting health and progress.

Do you need to go that far in order to lose weight and get healthier? Not necessarily. But the information and experience that I picked up over the past five years while guiding patients through my protocols are now streamlined into the book you're holding and the four-week program you will learn. This is the foundation for *Women, Food, and Hormones.*

## NOT A ONE-SIZE-FITS-ALL PROGRAM

As described by the medical journal *The Lancet,* we are witnessing an "overabundance of information — some accurate and some not — that makes it harder for people to find trustworthy sources and reliable guidance when needed."[3] Unproved theories and so-called miracle cures contribute to today's infodemic, the flood of misinformation regarding the reasons for our obesity epidemic and the metabolic catastrophe following in its wake. The situation is complicated by the fact that diet programs don't work the same way for every person and that many such programs have been created by men and tested on male bodies, not female ones.

The fact that you have a unique biology can get lost in the media hype around the latest diet craze. Bear with me for a quick "science moment." Let's consider the diet trend now most frequently searched for online. This is the ketogenic diet — or "keto," as it has been affectionately nicknamed — a very low carbohydrate diet that puts the body in a state of ketosis, which means it is burning fat instead of sugar. Very few authors of books promoting the keto diet or its practitioners are paying attention to the contradictory outcomes reported by researchers. For example, the diet may not be the best choice for some people at risk for cancer or already battling it.[4] According to limited studies, ketones produced by the body when on a ketogenic diet may be associated with progression of cancer, metastasis, and poor clinical outcomes.[5]

Based on the scientific data, the ketogenic diet is not a one-size-fits-all quick fix. It's more of a mixed bag: On classic keto, some women lose weight. Some develop better focus, or perhaps avoid certain types of cancer. On the other hand, some women develop thyroid dysfunction. Some find the diet physically stressful, though they may not consciously notice this; nonetheless, stress-related hormones may block weight loss. For just under half of the women on a ketogenic diet, changes to menstrual hormones and loss of the monthly cycle occur; the quality of studies reporting these results is, however, uneven. Some women actually *gain* weight on diets like keto, and for the most part, no one is warning them about the effects on hormones.

Given this range of results—from the impressive to the potentially harmful—anyone considering a ketogenic diet needs to have a medical doctor in her court. We need medical doctors to make sense of the contradictory information, to help women follow protocols proven to work, and to keep them safe.

## AN ANTIDOTE TO THE INFODEMIC

I am a physician-scientist who practices precision medicine. I am a clinical assistant professor of integrative medicine and nutritional sciences at Sidney Kimmel Medical College, Thomas Jefferson University, located in Philadelphia, Pennsylvania. There I also serve as the director of precision medicine at the Marcus Institute of Integrative Health.

In *Women, Food, and Hormones,* I will teach you the scientific basis of hormone balancing by changing what, how, and when you eat, using the Gottfried Protocol. You'll see hundreds of citations from peer-reviewed journals to document my statements about the key hormones of metabolism—you will meet them all shortly.

But I'm getting ahead of myself. You'll get to know the names and functions of the key hormones very soon, and how they work together to create an extraordinary symphony in your body—or deafening alarm bells. Learning how each instrument, each hormone, works and what you can do to encourage the beautiful music that comes from balanced hormones is so empowering. When your hormones work in harmony, you won't just look better—you'll also feel better.

If you go to a conventional doctor for treatment of symptoms of hormone imbalance, you will likely receive a prescription for a pill. The doctor may try to tell you that lifestyle changes aren't enough. But that's not what I've found. In fact, as a leader in the integrative, precision, and functional medicine movement, I believe that lifestyle changes are the best hope for a comprehensive solution. Lifestyle choices, starting with food, play a huge role in hormonal balance, and by extension, your total health. In this book, you'll be learning more about the latest scientific breakthroughs concerning hormones and your health. You'll find out how to reset your hormones with your fork and glass in Part 2, which covers the how-to of the Gottfried Protocol.

The Gottfried Protocol is not some fad diet, but rather a science-based approach to health for women. If you've read my previous books, you know that I'm not easily sold on the latest trends. In *Brain Body Diet,* I question the keto diet's value as a weight-loss plan for women. Since writing *Brain Body Diet,* I've pored over the studies published on the subject each year. After two failed attempts at trying to follow keto the classic way, I came up with an approach that worked for me and can work for most women. Then I taught my patients how to do it and watched hundreds of them achieve their weight-loss goals and sustain a healthy weight by using a modified ketogenic diet paired with designed support detoxification and fasting. My approach takes into account individual differences and female physiology.

Throughout this book, I provide general advice that has worked for many of my patients. But not everyone is the same. A ketogenic diet, the supplements I recommend, or other aspects of the system I suggest here may not be appropriate for women (or men) who have certain medical conditions, medical histories, or unique sensitivities.

And of course I cannot give individualized medical advice in this book. It's never a bad idea when starting a new diet or health plan to talk with your physician and health team to make sure the plan is right for you.

## WHY IT'S NOT THE SAME FOR WOMEN

Even though women are more likely than men to carry some extra pounds with no health risks, women face more societal pressure to be thin. In my medical practice, I've seen the private suffering of women of all shapes, sizes, races, and ethnicities who struggle to meet our culture's unrealistic standards when it comes to weight. I've learned that even women who aren't overweight are often battling body-image issues and unhealthy relationships with food.

I want you to know that anyone, regardless of body type, can be healthy and strong and feel energized. While many men and women turn to keto, for example, because they are hoping to lose weight, I believe the goal should be health, not weight loss for the sake of weight loss. Nevertheless, we have to wonder why women's bodies respond to food differently than men's do.

In this book, I expose the keto paradox: Why does classic keto help men lose weight and cause some women to gain it? Why does classic keto reverse some diseases and exacerbate others? When does keto clear inflammation, and when does keto cause it? I keep finding the same answer: *hormones!*

High-fat, low-carbohydrate diets cause weight loss for many reasons, but probably not quite in the way you're thinking. Many people think, *If I go keto, I can eat lots of satisfying fat, lose weight, and fit into that cute dress I wore in college.* Well, maybe. The classic ketogenic diet, as practiced most commonly today, doesn't work for many women (and the cute dress stays in storage) because the ketogenic process is misunderstood and therefore not managed for success. Most people think that a low-carb diet causes weight loss simply because eating fewer carbs reduces insulin levels and burns fat. If it worked like that, switching from regular soda to diet soda would cause weight loss, but it doesn't; if you replace one hormonal calamity (sugar) with a potentially worse one (artificial sweeteners), your hormonal messaging gets thrown further out of whack. A common result of switching to diet soda is weight *gain*.[6] Furthermore, if you starve your body of carbohydrates over the long term, you may lose weight, but unfortunately this may cause additional problems, ones that have given the classic keto diet a bad rap.

I have seen up close the frustration the classic keto diet can cause. I meet a large number of "keto refugees" in my office and in my online courses. Some women are too stressed to perform classic keto successfully (stress affects hormones, as discussed on page 30), or they don't get the carbohydrates they need to promote normal hormonal regulation. They gained weight on keto, or didn't lose weight, or started to doubt the high-animal-fat and high-calorie food plan. They've experienced more inflammation and more mood crashes, and they even whisper about the dreaded keto crotch (if you need to ask what that is, consider yourself lucky). They are wondering why butter in their coffee and fat bombs (a popular keto dessert) aren't making them feel or look great, although their husbands or their male co-workers claim success with them.

The truth is, classic keto has mostly been studied in men, and it needs to be modified for many women in order to be successful.

We aren't totally sure why women respond to keto differently.[7] But experts have some ideas. Hormones play a primary role. There's the stress gap — the fact that women are twice as likely to suffer from stress, anxiety, and depression. Women more commonly experience thyroid problems and autoimmunity. Women are more sensitive to carbohydrate restriction and calorie restriction than men are; these restrictions may activate an alarm that shuts down menstruation and increases inflammation — and may explain why so many women on keto lose menstrual regularity. Experts suggest that, compared to men, women are more likely to experience a plummet in blood sugar. Maybe a combination of these issues causes the problem.

There is one thing we know for sure: your hormones dictate your success or lack thereof on the classic ketogenic diet. You won't see the results you want if you don't factor hormones into the equation. I go into more depth about these hormones — and include questionnaires to help you determine whether your hormones are in balance — in Part 1.

We all have these hormones. We may have different levels at one age versus another, or one woman may have more or less compared to another. These hormones juggle function a bit differently (for instance, you need both growth hormone and testosterone for bone strength, but they strengthen the bone in different ways), but all of them are influenced by what we eat.

For example, studies show that higher fat in the diet, and polyunsaturated fatty acids specifically (the fat found in many nuts, flaxseed, and fish), contributes to increased concentration of testosterone in women. (More details are in the Notes.)[8] Once again there is a gap in the research: the effect of the ketogenic diet on testosterone has not yet been studied in healthy women.

When losing weight, men have something known as the *testosterone advantage.* Because their testosterone levels are typically ten times higher than those of women and testosterone is responsible for increasing muscle mass, men have more muscle and burn calories faster. When they diet, using the keto plan or something else, men tend to lose weight faster than women. Only for men has the ketogenic diet been shown to raise testosterone, improve lean body mass, and decrease fat mass.[9] In other words, men may get a double testosterone advantage with classic keto. They start off with higher testosterone levels, then the ketogenic diet and the resulting boost to testosterone help them burn more fat and build more muscle, so they drop weight and look better faster.

While higher levels of testosterone may give men an edge, lower testosterone and higher estrogen levels may put some women at a disadvantage and lead to slower or lower results. On the other hand, estrogen has many positive influences on the body, no matter a woman's age. It is the main reason why we have a lower rate of heart disease than men do before age fifty-two, and why we tend to store fat around our hips and thighs, a far healthier place than the waist for these reserves. Fortunately, you don't need to know your exact levels of these hormones, unless you prefer that level of precision. I will guide you, based on your questionnaire results, to customize the protocol so that it works for you.

## HOW I CAN HELP YOU, WOMAN TO WOMAN

The Gottfried Protocol is designed to sidestep the keto paradox with a program that's tailor-made for a woman's body. You will be able to sustain a lower weight while eating a healthy quantity of high-quality carbs, resulting in better hormone balance and more fat loss.

We all need help. This book is designed to help you reconnect your food with your hormones so you feel whole and at peace with your body and your food: no longer at war, no longer feeling flabby or sluggish and wondering why nothing works. The strategies and case studies in this book are body positive. The goal is not to get skinny but rather to regain the healthiest possible version of you. It works, if you do it right. And there's rigorous science behind it.

My promise: I'll put *science first* to help keep you safe. I'll help you decide whether the Gottfried Protocol is right for you, and whether you'll need a few personal workarounds to ensure success. I won't tell you to eat fake food that works over the short term but doesn't create long-term freedom around food and a healthy gut, and I won't advise anything that is not supported by good evidence. I'll assist you in determining your carb threshold, or how long your leash needs to be — each day, each week, each month — so that you can have a piece of cake at your son's birthday party and occasionally enjoy a splurge when at a dinner party with friends. I'll help you avoid the yo-yo roller-coaster of weight loss and regain that plagues many women.

Keeping you informed and safe is not a promise I take lightly. This is not a pledge to get you skinny in one week, with no effort on your part. That's a potentially dangerous fantasy.

Instead, I will give you easy-to-implement tools to customize the Gottfried Protocol for your own body, so that you can achieve all the benefits: burn fat, reduce inflammation, fight cancer, balance hormones and gut bacteria, improve neurological diseases, and even increase life span. I am offering you a proven solution, supported by research and hundreds of success stories, mine included.

## MEET THE HORMONES

In this book, you will discover a new way to eat for your hormones. Hormones decide what the body does with the fuel you eat. Your hormones exist in delicate balance, playing alongside one another like instruments in an orchestra. Throughout the day, your hormones fluctuate in rhythm, going up and down like crescendos in a symphony. Each hormone is like a specific instrument that must play on time, at the right volume, and in the correct cadence. In combination, your hormones create a beautiful harmony, which serves as your stable sense of well-being and grace.

What are the hormones of metabolism? Thousands have been detected and researched, but the key hormones we'll focus on are insulin, cortisol, leptin, ghrelin, thyroid, estrogen, testosterone, and growth hormone. Metabolic hormones are involved in thousands of micro communications and processes in the body. To name a few, hormones are involved in satiety (leptin, insulin), hunger (ghrelin, cortisol), female qualities (estradiol), more masculine qualities (testosterone, the most abundant hormone in women, and involved in vitality, muscle mass, and agency), and fat burning (insulin, growth hormone, and cortisol). These are the hormones that govern your response to food, but the relationship is bidirectional.

Metabolic hormones regulate your response to food, and in turn, food regulates metabolic hormones. Insulin is the most influential. It's like a bouncer at a club that either opens the door to glucose or not. If the bouncer doesn't open the door to usher in the glucose, the glucose in your blood rises and over time can lead to insulin block and fat accumulation. That's the central problem of insulin resistance, and it can be identified way before a diagnosis of diabetes.

We won't get mired in explaining every hormone in detail, as it's not necessary to get the Gottfried Protocol to work for you. What's important to know is that these hormones are at work in the background, either helping you lose weight and feel great, or not.

Writing about hormones is about telling the truth, especially the difficult truths about being female and over the age of thirty-five. The levels of many hormones start to drop in our twenties (testosterone, DHEA), thirties (growth hormone, progesterone), and forties through fifties (estrogen). At the same time, other key metabolic hormones, insulin and leptin (and its cousin, ghrelin, the hunger hormone), can rise. These combined hormonal shifts can make life feel more difficult. Why?

- Metabolism slows down yet appetite increases, which means belly fat accumulates seemingly overnight, increasing inflammation. Your weight climbs.
- The liver, the primary organ that regulates fat loss, loses reserve. It is busy metabolizing hormones, clearing toxins, dealing with your latest alcoholic beverage, adjusting cholesterol levels, trying to sort out what fuel you are eating now (carbs? protein? fat?), and generally trying to run the show for the rest of the body.
- The rest of the gut, including the intestines, suffers too. Your gut is involved in regulating your hormones. Most of my patients have one or more problems with their gut that can impede fat loss, such as an imbalance of gut microbes (dysbiosis) or leaky gut syndrome (increased intestinal permeability, which can occur when the tight junctions between the cells lining the small intestine become disrupted).
- On a related note, most of my patients have a substantial *fiber gap*. What you eat has a major influence on the microbes in your gut, a relationship known as the host-microbe interaction. You need the right prebiotic fibers to feed the benevolent bugs, thereby improving immune function and hormone balance. You may not be getting enough of these key fibers.[10]

When you follow the Gottfried Protocol, you'll specifically address each of these challenges, from metabolism to gut health. Your healthy population of gut microbes will increase, and we'll say good-bye to the ones that may be hanging on to fat and inflammation.

## WHAT IS THE GOTTFRIED PROTOCOL?

The hormone-balancing Gottfried Protocol has three tenets: detox-ification, nutritional ketosis, and intermittent fasting. After experi-menting with the Gottfried Protocol for the past five years, I've dis-covered the essential sequence of these three tenets to activate fat loss for women over the age of thirty-five.

- **Detoxification.** Activating your body's detoxification pathways is essential to prevent the problems that women commonly experience in ketosis, so we do that first. Why? Detoxification clears out your liver and eliminates any recirculating, tired hormones that are clogging up your metabolism.
- **Nutritional ketosis.** You enter nutritional ketosis when you follow a food plan that is low in carbohydrates, moderate in protein, and high in fat. I have adjusted the classic ketogenic diet to make it more effective at restoring insulin levels in women and helping you lose weight. To cut a long story short, you will be (1) eating more plants; (2) consuming tablespoons of extra-virgin olive oil, the occasional spoonful of medium-chain triglyceride oil (associated with weight loss, improved satiety, and removal of alcohol), prebiotics, and probiotics; and (3) tracking net carbs, among other macronutrients. You will use your macronutrients to calculate your ketogenic ratio, and then measure your glucose-ketone ratio (more about this in Part 2). Success on a ketogenic diet is multifaceted — part of it is psychological. The diet's fat-burning power often results in weight loss, improved lean body mass, and increased metabolic rate in a short time, which in turn inspires continuing adherence to the plan and then more improved outcomes. Nonetheless, pitfalls exist, and I will teach you how to avoid them. (See page 18 for a graphic illustrating how the ketogenic diet works.)

- **Intermittent fasting.** This type of fasting means you don't eat for twelve to twenty-four hours in a single day. Data show that intermittent fasting is particularly effective at encouraging weight loss because it improves the balance of many hormones (including insulin, ghrelin, leptin, and afternoon cortisol) and leads to metabolic switching, as reviewed recently in the venerable *New England Journal of Medicine.*[11] (Metabolic switching is when you use fasting and other techniques to suppress insulin and glucose to a level that triggers a switch from burning carbohydrates to burning fat in the body.) Fasting helps regulate inflammation, increases brain function so you feel sharper, lowers blood pressure, and may modulate leptin so you feel more satisfied.[12] Still not convinced? Intermittent fasting helps with cholesterol levels (see details in the Notes).[13] Perhaps most important, I've found intermittent fasting to be extremely effective in aiding women over the age of thirty-five to lose fat and feel better; about 95 percent of my patients are successful at it.

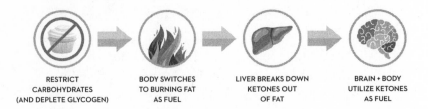

| RESTRICT CARBOHYDRATES (AND DEPLETE GLYCOGEN) | BODY SWITCHES TO BURNING FAT AS FUEL | LIVER BREAKS DOWN KETONES OUT OF FAT | BRAIN + BODY UTILIZE KETONES AS FUEL |

## WHY METABOLIC FLEXIBILITY MATTERS TO YOU

Earlier, I defined metabolism as the sum total of chemical reactions that determine how you feel and the speed with which you burn fuel. Understanding the speed of your metabolism is important, but another significant yet often overlooked aspect of metabolism is its *flexibility.* Before you start restricting carbs and deprive yourself perhaps unnecessarily, find out how metabolically flexible you are. Carbs are not the enemy, but lack of metabolic flexibility just might be.

What is metabolic flexibility? It's the ability to adapt to changes in metabolic demand,[14] like when you eat an apple (rich in healthy carbohydrates) versus a slab of salmon (rich in healthy fat), or when you go for sixteen hours without eating and your body needs to burn fat to create fuel. If you have diabetes, are obese, or have an "apple-shaped" body, with more fat at the waist than the hips, then it's likely you have metabolic inflexibility. Metabolic flexibility exists on a spectrum, ranging from normal metabolic flexibility to inflexibility. Indicators that inflexibility is setting in include rising blood-glucose levels, insulin resistance (when insulin starts to rise in the blood), prediabetes, early damage to blood vessels, abnormal lipids, hypertension, and obesity.

Metabolic inflexibility is a major issue affecting many people: according to the Centers for Disease Control, obesity rates continue to rise.[15] Up to 38 percent of the US population has prediabetes.[16] Even people with a normal weight, or who are overweight but not obese, might have metabolic inflexibility. (This doesn't just affect how you fit into your clothes; excess weight is linked to difficulty in fighting illnesses like coronavirus and may make you less responsive to vaccination.[17]) The good news is that if you are metabolically inflexible, or on your way to inflexibility, we can reverse the condition with precision medicine to improve the way you eat, move, think, and sleep.

The Gottfried Protocol will put you on the path to metabolic flexibility: low fasting blood sugar after an overnight fast and mild ketosis from producing a small amount of ketones (a sign that you are burning fat), normal blood sugar after eating, and a normal waist-to-hip ratio. You won't crave the crappy carbs anymore. In short, food freedom!

## YOU ARE NEVER A LOST CAUSE

You are never too old to balance your hormones. Yet on social media and elsewhere, I hear women say, "I'm in menopause — it's too late for me." Not true. Many of the hormones addressed, especially insulin, growth hormone, testosterone, and estrogen, are modulated by food, detoxification, ketosis, and timing of meals. There is no upper limit on the best age to achieve hormonal balance.

Similarly, you are never a lost cause. Even if you've been frustrated by a lack of results and feel like your metabolism is the slowest of your life, you can still make progress — I have the case studies to prove it — though it may take longer. You might lose a pound per day initially, like Lara, age forty-five, did in the first five days, or more slowly, like Lotus, age fifty-one — but Lotus now has lost 39 pounds, even though she had a slow metabolism at the start of the Gottfried Protocol. Keep the long view.

Fortunately, you can successfully follow the evidence-based Gottfried Protocol, get your metabolic hormones back on track, and lose weight regardless of whether you are omnivore, pescatarian, vegetarian, or vegan.[18] I've included recipes and sample meal plans to mix and match, so that you can hit your daily targets and be triumphant.

If you chase symptoms with medication, you are less likely to heal than if you chart a new path with the lifestyle medicine of the Gottfried Protocol. You can wipe the slate clean and create hormonal homeostasis. You'll come to love and value your body in a whole new way, and you'll be inspired to eat this way because you feel so good and your health problems resolve. Baggage, trauma, and self-sabotage will become a thing of the past.

## LET'S ADD LIFE TO YOUR YEARS

Losing fat after age thirty-five is not about discipline so much as *what to eat, when to eat it, and how your food talks to your hormones.* Most people don't realize that hormones drive metabolism. When your hormones start to get imbalanced after age thirty-five, following certain rules will help you avoid a thickening waist and greater risk of heart disease, diabetes, and cancer. I'll share with you more about my story in Chapter 1, and throughout the book, you'll meet other women who've followed the Gottfried Protocol, encountered a new way to eat in order to feed their hormones, and experienced fat and weight loss.

I'll give you a proven way to enter mild ketosis that will activate your get-me-lean hormones, reverse inflammation, and give you peace of mind. The Gottfried Protocol is based on my own small clinical study with ten overweight and obese women before and after following a ketogenic diet. I used a personalized approach with an N-of-1 design, which arguably produces the highest-quality scientific evidence. In this method of doing research, each individual is the focus of a separate case study. [19]

When you learn the basics of what to eat and when, and how your food talks to your hormones, you can create a hormonal symphony that makes you feel energized throughout the day, without those 4 p.m. dips. You'll burn fat instead of storing it at your waist, where it increases your risk for most chronic diseases. You'll fit into your clothes, so that picking an outfit will take ten seconds, not ten hours —because all of your clothes will look great. You'll feel physically, psychologically, and emotionally satisfied, so you won't eat two dinners every night because you feel like you deserve it. You'll have more time for the things you love. You will learn to eat in a manner that works for your hormones, that connects the dots between nutrition and hormones for your body, and that adds way more life to your years.

# 1

---

# THE TRUTH ABOUT WOMEN, HORMONES, AND WEIGHT

*Grant me the serenity to accept*
*the hormones I cannot change,*
*the courage to change the ones I can,*
*and the wisdom to tell the difference.*

I call this the Serenity Prayer for Hormones. Why invoke a prayer? If you've ever experienced hormone-induced weight gain, inexplicably gained 5 pounds right before your period, or suffered from PMS or sleepless nights, thanks to shifting hormones, then you probably understand.

Our hormones rule our bodies, dictating how we think, feel, and look. And while I can't turn back the clock to give you the hormones you had in your early twenties (and the fast metabolism that came with them), the good news is that we have science-based guidelines to bring key hormones back into balance. My goal with this book is to empower you to do so. And that's what the Serenity Prayer for Hormones is all about.

I learned the hard way that people, particularly women, with endocrine dysfunction — a hormone imbalance known for certain common signs and symptoms — tend to struggle the most with their weight. These are my patients with the most stubborn weight-loss resistance. Throughout the book, you'll hear stories about them and my online followers and how they were able to turn frustration into success. I suspect you'll relate to more than a few.

The good news is that we can do something about it too, starting with your fork. We now know what works to resolve hormone imbalances, especially in women over the age of thirty-five. The key is to begin with food, because what you eat is the backbone of every hormone you make. Your food choices may seem inconsequential in the moment, but every bite determines the balance of hormones, the health of your gut and nervous system, the function of your blood vessels, and the strength of your immune system.

Here is the Serenity Prayer in action:

Melissa and I were in my medical office, reviewing her hormone tests. Melissa reported subtle changes in her periods, which suggested she had begun the perimenopausal transition. At age thirty-eight, Melissa was about 30 pounds overweight, with a waist circumference of 40 inches, and she told me she had tried absolutely everything to lose weight. She looked me straight in the eye and said, "Just tell it to me straight. Explain *what I can change* and *what I can't* with my hormones. I know that as I get older, there's a limit to how much I can course-correct. If I make the changes you suggest, will I lose weight? Do I have hormone issues that are beyond repair?" She sighed heavily for the second time.

No! Your hormones are not beyond repair. Like most patients in my practice who are overweight, obese, or just have to work incredibly hard to maintain a healthy weight, Melissa struggles with hormone imbalances. (The telltale physical sign for Melissa, besides the changes in her period, was her apple shape—a common term for larger midsections, with a waist circumference divided by hip circumference that is above 0.85. In Melissa's case, her waist-to-hip ratio was 0.92.) After a round of medical detective work, we found problems with insulin and thyroid—two of the most common hormone imbalances that make it hard to lose weight. In my experience, insulin is the worst, but thyroid and sex hormones are close behind and interrelated.

For the third time, Melissa sighed heavily. According to Chinese traditional medicine, this is a sign of liver qi (pronounced "chee") stagnation, and to my mind, a clue that her hormones were not in balance.

---

## The Liver, Hormones, and Traditional Chinese Medicine

Though I'm not a practitioner of traditional Chinese medicine (TCM), I've learned a lot over the years from studying its ancient precepts. According to TCM, liver qi stagnation (LQS) is often linked to all sorts of hormonal imbalance, beginning with premenstrual syndrome and irregular cycles, but by the time a woman reaches perimenopause, there are likely several patterns at play. The liver in TCM is defined by function and is not equivalent to the anatomical organ known in Western medicine as the liver. The life force of the liver, known as qi, can stagnate as a result of stress or anxiety. When qi flows properly, things are in harmony and function properly, but when flow is blocked, problems occur.

Liver qi is responsible for movement of qi through the body, so when it becomes stagnant, women may experience mood swings, frustration that erupts easily, constipation, premenstrual syndrome, and irregular periods, among other problems. (Learn more about what my acupuncturist, Emily Hooker, has to say about liver qi stagnation in the Notes.)[1]

---

Do you struggle with hormone imbalance affecting your weight? Take the following questionnaire to see.

## Metabolic Hormone Questionnaire

Do you have or have you experienced any of the following symptoms in the past six months?

- Have you been steadily gaining weight since the birth of a child, perimenopause, or menopause?
- Do you experience high stress or chronic low-grade stress? Sweat the small stuff?
- Do you have high blood pressure, now defined as systolic blood pressure greater than 120 or diastolic blood pressure over 80?[2]
- Is your body mass index 25 or higher? Use an online calculator to determine your BMI, or use this formula: BMI = weight ÷ height$^2$. If you used kilograms and centimeters, you have your result. If you used pounds and inches, you need to multiply the result by 703. For example, for a woman who is 150 pounds with a height of 64 inches, BMI = (150 ÷ 64$^2$) × 703 = 25.7.
- Have you ever gained 3 to 5 pounds overnight? Or 5 to 7 pounds with menstruation?
- Are you fatigued at any point during the day, despite adequate rest?
- Do you notice thinning head hair, loss of outer third of eyebrows, puffy face, dry and coarse skin, constipation, lack of energy, intolerance of cold, infertility, heavy menstruation, carpal tunnel syndrome, or any combination of these?
- Do you feel like something blocks you from losing weight, no matter what you try?
- Do you struggle to adhere to a diet? As in, you know what to do but you cannot stick to a plan over the long run, and so you lose the same 5 to 10 pounds over and over again?
- Do you eat very clean but don't feel that the bathroom scale reflects it?

- Do you experience food cravings, particularly for sweets, chocolate, cheese, or bread?
- Have you tried a strict ketogenic diet, but it didn't work for you? You didn't lose the weight as expected, you didn't experience mental clarity, you hit a plateau, or you gained weight?
- Do you have a diagnosis of Hashimoto's thyroiditis, celiac disease, rheumatoid arthritis, multiple sclerosis, systemic lupus erythematosus, psoriasis, or some other autoimmune disease?
- Has your appetite increased? Do you find yourself still hungry after a normal-sized serving of food that previously satisfied you?
- Has your blood sugar been rising? Is your fasting blood sugar greater than 85 mg/dL, which I consider out of the optimal zone? Or is it greater than 99 mg/dL, in the prediabetes or diabetes range, based on tests taken by your health-care practitioner?
- Have you experienced more difficulty sleeping through the night since giving birth or perimenopause, are you feeling more stress, or all of the above?
- Do you have extra fat in your abdomen? Is your waist circumference greater than 35 inches for women, or greater than 40 inches for men? (Another way to measure it is a waist-to-hip ratio greater than 0.85 in women, or greater than 0.90 in men.)
- Examine the skin around your neck and where you have folds in the skin, such as your axilla (armpits). Do you see darkening of the skin and a velvet-like texture, known as acanthosis nigricans?

### Interpreting Your Score

If you answered yes to five or more of the questions above, you probably have a hormone imbalance affecting your weight and metabolism. If this is you, don't panic. First of all, you're not alone. My practice is full of women with hormone imbalances. Overall, about 80 percent of them score 5 or higher, and lab testing confirms that one or more metabolic hormones are out of balance. My personal score was 10 before I designed the Gottfried Protocol for metabolic hormones, so if your score is high, don't fret.

Fortunately, you found this book. My goal is to identify the root cause of your imbalance and resolve it. (If you are experiencing excessive or severe symptoms, be sure to consult a health-care practitioner.) Continue reading this chapter to learn more about the connection between hormones and weight gain, and how to optimize diet to achieve weight loss.

# FIVE PRINCIPLES
# OF WOMEN + WEIGHT

In my late thirties, I gave birth to my second daughter and my hormones went crazy. I lost my ability to manage my weight easily. In hindsight, this was probably caused by a combination of toxic stress, my borderline blood sugar issues during pregnancy, the demands of motherhood, and getting older. But the experience shifted my career from general OB/GYN to precision medicine, with emphasis on understanding the intersection of women, hormones, and weight. Not every woman goes through a period of crazy hormones, but many do.

As I mentioned in the introduction, your hormones are like your own internal symphony orchestra, playing music to your cells 24/7. If your inner song is in rhythm and harmony, you'll be resilient and metabolically flexible. Or, if it's like mine at age thirty-nine, it can sound like noise: the clarinet is too soft, the cello is too loud, and the beat is off. It may seem like you're doing everything right with your diet and workouts, but the results don't show. Conducting the symphony may seem to be out of your control, but the truth is, you have more power than you realize to bring your hormones into harmony by changing your lifestyle.

Here are the five principles I discovered that will keep your hormonal symphony in tune.

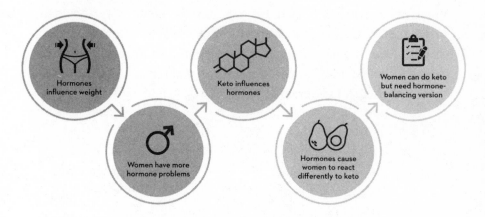

1. Hormones influence weight.
2. Women have more hormone problems than men do.
3. The ketogenic diet influences hormones.
4. Because of their hormones, women react differently to the ketogenic diet than men do.
5. Women can follow a ketogenic diet, but they do better with a hormone-balancing version, such as the Gottfried Protocol.

I will walk you through the details of each of these principles so that you can get your hormones back on beat and holding it all together—and lose weight for good.

## 1. Hormones influence weight.

Several hormones are involved in the control of weight, fluid retention, and the amount of fat carried on the body. It's the fat, particularly visceral fat at your waist, that concerns me most. In this section, I want to connect the dots between your fat, your hormones, and your health once and for all.

Which hormones? The list is long: insulin, cortisol, thyroid, testosterone, estrogen, progesterone, growth hormone, and leptin. (The diagram below details several of these hormones and where they are produced in the endocrine system, the set of glands that produces the various hormones that circulate throughout your body.) The hormone imbalance that rises to the top is insulin block (also known as insulin resistance), which causes the body's cells to become numb to insulin. Then the pancreas needs to make more and more insulin to do the job of pushing glucose into cells. Insulin block is closely tied to weight gain and visceral fat.[3]

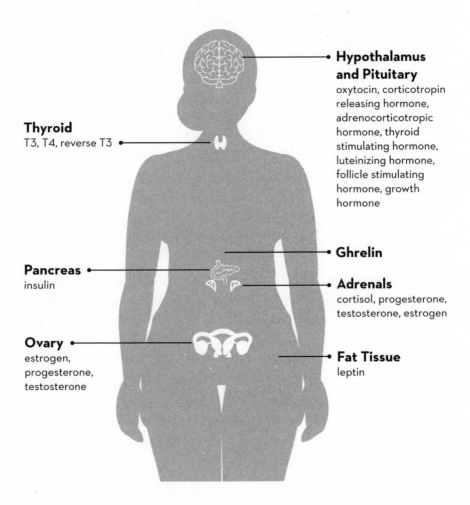

**Hypothalamus and Pituitary**
oxytocin, corticotropin releasing hormone, adrenocorticotropic hormone, thyroid stimulating hormone, luteinizing hormone, follicle stimulating hormone, growth hormone

**Thyroid**
T3, T4, reverse T3

**Ghrelin**

**Pancreas**
insulin

**Adrenals**
cortisol, progesterone, testosterone, estrogen

**Ovary**
estrogen, progesterone, testosterone

**Fat Tissue**
leptin

Hormones are chemical messengers — think of them as text messages sent around your body. They request certain functions, like stabilizing your mood, making your skin moist, building muscle at the gym, and telling you to eat more. When they are in order, you can reach a healthy weight and maintain it. You can sleep well at night and wake up refreshed. You don't feel cranky, anxious, and fat.

Back to the symphony analogy for hormones — the official conductor of the orchestra is your brain, particularly the parts known as the hypothalamus and the pituitary gland. Your brain communicates to your other endocrine organs, like your adrenal glands (brass), ovaries (testes in men; woodwinds), thyroid (percussion), and fat (strings). But the conductor is vulnerable. Poor eating, too much drinking, and excess stress will affect its function.

When the conductor is on top of its game, well fed and resilient, hormones remain in balance and the music is wonderful. Your usual strategies for weight loss will tend to work, just as I found was the case early in my thirties, before I had kids. When the conductor is off kilter, so are your hormones. They may individually conspire against weight loss, and even cross-talk to make matters worse. For example, Melissa's thyroid problems didn't occur in isolation. Her elevated insulin levels and fat deposits made her thyroid function worse.[4] Then, to make matters more unfair, being overweight increased her chances of developing more thyroid problems.[5] Fortunately, the Gottfried Protocol helps your brain conduct the symphony with ease and grace, so your body can return to a state of balance and health.

There are many common endocrine problems that lead to *weight-loss resistance*, including thyroid imbalances and insulin block, and they can be caused by a myriad of factors, including high stress and chemicals in the environment — found in body products, cleaning supplies, and food — that disrupt specific hormones. Plus, what you eat can affect your hormones, as we'll discuss in the next chapter.

## 2. Women have more hormone
## problems than men do.

Straight talk: compared to men, women have more hormone imbalances, leading to higher rates of anxiety, depression, and insomnia.[6] The unpleasant symptoms of hormone imbalance create a cascade of additional problems, particularly when it comes to weight loss. For example, sleeping less than six hours or more than nine is associated with metabolic syndrome, a constellation of belly fat, insulin block, blood sugar problems, high blood pressure, and lipid issues.[7]

As a physician and a woman, I'm all too familiar with the vicious cycle of body dissatisfaction, stress, and weight gain. Women who struggle with extra weight, even a small number of pounds, often find themselves locked in a battle with their body. Maybe you can relate? It's no wonder women experience more body dissatisfaction than men do. In advertisements, media such as TV programs and movies, and well-intended comments from family members and friends, we're told from a young age that we need to be thin and beautiful, no matter the cost.

When we are socialized to internalize this ideal, we do a thing that academics call *self-objectification,* making us more likely to experience body shame and dissatisfaction. This means we internalize an observer's view of our body as an object that must be evaluated on the basis of our looks, resulting in frequent and habitual monitoring of our outward appearance.[8] Women are more likely than men to do this. Women who self-objectify are more likely to have disordered eating.[9] Objectification sells products,[10] but self-objectification has a higher cost; that is, the internal battle that so many of my female patients experience.

In a sad, ironic twist, this self-objectification can lead to higher stress levels, even more hormone imbalance, and then weight gain. Many of my patients feel like they are more stressed than ever — and they aren't alone. Women experience higher levels of stress than men do, as shown in the American Psychological Association's annual stress survey. In 2020, it was reported that more women than men feel that now is the lowest point in the country's history that they can remember. (Maybe men are paying less attention?)

This stress affects our health—and our hormones. Most women are unaware of their hormone imbalances. But even before menopause, women are more vulnerable to them. The most common endocrine disorders affecting women before menopause are problems with testosterone, insulin, and thyroid.[11] The most common cause of hypothyroidism in the United States is Hashimoto's thyroiditis, an autoimmune disease that is *five to ten times* more common in women than men.

Then additional hormonal shifts come with age and menopause, when women more commonly experience low estrogen, testosterone, and growth hormone. Since estrogen is involved in many activities, including appetite arousal and food intake,[12] loss of hormones like estrogen can trigger weight gain. The main estrogen that regulates the female body is estradiol. See the illustration for how estrogen changes as women age, leading to wild fluctuations in perimenopause that can increase appetite.

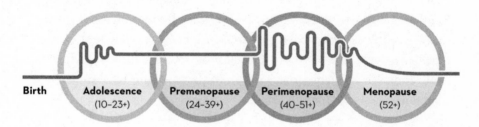

| Birth | Adolescence (10–23+) | Premenopause (24–39+) | Perimenopause (40–51+) | Menopause (52+) |

On the other hand, when overweight or obese women lose fat, growth hormone increases.[13] The good news is that you set off a virtuous cycle: you are more able to recover after exercise, heal from an injury, boost metabolism, and then you burn more fat, and growth hormone rises more. Success!

Just knowing that hormones can block weight loss, and that women are more likely to experience hormone imbalance, is part of the solution. And my protocol is designed to bring your hormones back into balance with a modified ketogenic diet.

### 3. The ketogenic diet influences hormones.

Here's what's good about the keto diet—a low-carbohydrate, moderate-protein, high-fat diet—when it comes to hormones. It is one of the most effective strategies to repair insulin, the main hormone involved in weight gain, general misery, and cardiovascular disease, which is the number-one killer of both men and women.

The trouble is that keto has the potential to adversely affect other hormones, including cortisol, thyroid, and estrogen. Chronic elevations in cortisol are associated with lots of problems, including oxidative stress (the rust of aging that accumulates in our cells), cholesterol problems, poor vascular function, platelet clumping, plaque buildup in the arteries[14]—and increased visceral fat, the problem I worry about the most, in terms of your health.[15] In men, consuming carbohydrates reduces cortisol production.[16] Likewise, restricting carbs may *increase* cortisol production, unless you know how to avoid it.

Estrogen may get out of balance in people who eat a "lazy keto" diet, like fast-food burgers wrapped in lettuce with bacon on top, and forget to eat sufficient vegetables to feed good microbes in the gut. Healthy estrogen balance relies on a healthy ecosystem of microbes. People who eat more animal products, like meat and cheese, but skimp on vegetables risk a rise in the levels of misbehaving members of the estrogen family.

### 4. Because of their hormones, women react differently to classic keto than men do.

We've already talked about the keto paradox, so you know that the traditional keto diet doesn't always work for women. We still need more studies that explore how keto influences women's hormones, but some possible reasons for differences in outcomes have arisen in the research.

First, keto may not provide enough carbs for women—carbs help mitigate the stress response, lower cortisol, boost growth hormone, and support thyroid function. Second, women and men also differ in terms of how and where their body fat is stored, in their hormonal production, and in their brain responses to signals regulating weight and distribution of body fat. Women tend to store energy as fat in the subcutaneous space under the skin, whereas men are more likely to store energy as fat in their belly. Think "hourglass" or "pear" figure versus "dad bod" and beer bellies. This is called *partitioning*—women tend to partition fat in their subcutaneous space and become fat in the lower body (hips, butt, thighs), and men partition fat in their abdomen, in and around their abdominal organs.

Men have 50 percent more lean body mass and 13 percent lower fat mass than premenopausal women do.[17] Men, perimenopausal women, and menopausal women accumulate more fat in their belly than premenopausal women do, resulting in an "apple" body shape and a greater risk of developing complications associated with obesity.[18] For premenopausal women, fat tends to be deposited in the lower body: the hips, butt, and thighs.[19] Starting in perimenopause, the period of time when menstruation changes as your ovaries run out of high-quality eggs, women become more like men in that they tend to store fat at the waist. As you'll learn in Chapter 5, when you take your own measurements, we want the waist-to-hip ratio to be less than 0.85 for women (and less than 0.90 for men). A high waist-to-hip ratio predicts a risk for many problems, including insulin resistance and heart attack.[20]

Third, when it comes to insulin and the risk of diabetes, men and women are different.[21] Overall, healthy premenopausal women are more sensitive to the hormone insulin than men are—that means we need lower amounts of insulin than men do to lower blood glucose levels. We have lower rates of metabolic syndrome, at least before menopause.[22] Unfortunately, our advantage over men disappears when blood glucose climbs.[23] That's the position I found myself in five years ago, as I started to enter perimenopause. For a variety of reasons involving stress and insufficient sleep, I stored more fat. It seemed like overnight my subcutaneous fat nearly doubled—especially on my hips and legs.

I developed prediabetes, with a fasting glucose between 100 and

125 mg/dL. As my visceral fat increased, I couldn't zip my jeans, a very sad affair that tends to kick off in perimenopause, as the body begins the transition to menopause, which usually starts at about age forty-seven. Estrogen levels decline, the rate of fat gain doubles, and lean body mass declines — these gains and losses continue until two years after the final menstrual period.[24] Changes in fat partitioning during perimenopause reflect hormonal changes in women, and are confirmed in animal models of menopause.[25] Body fat, waist circumference, and waist-to-hip ratio increase during the menopausal transition except in women who take hormone therapy.[26]

Alcohol consumption and exercise play an important role in weight gain for most women.[27] Applying the rule of partitioning, our fat deposits shift from making us hourglasses and pears to apples with more belly fat.[28] It's not just a problem of vanity: women gain an average of 5 pounds over three years of the menopausal transition, and 20 percent *gain 10 pounds or more.* No wonder I couldn't zip my jeans! The weight gain is associated with a greater risk of heart disease, high blood pressure, total cholesterol, low-density lipoprotein cholesterol, triglycerides, and fasting insulin.

Fourth, keto can also affect the thyroid gland. Some people develop thyroid problems such as lower triiodothyronine (T3) or thyroxine (T4) levels, which are suggestive but not diagnostic of hypothyroidism.[29] Many women feel the change as symptoms: constipation, cold hands and feet, and hair loss.[30] Given the risk of thyroid dysfunction with a classic keto diet, I recommend modifying keto with the Gottfried Protocol and having your thyroid levels checked every six months until further research clarifies the effects. Fortunately, I have not seen any thyroid issues arise with my protocol.

For people with epilepsy, following the classic ketogenic diet is associated with menstrual irregularity and constipation.[31] We do not know if the same is true for people without epilepsy on the ketogenic diet, though fecal volume (the amount of stool you produce) may decline. It may be especially important for women to keep their bowels moving regularly in order to obtain the benefits of keto, since regular bowel movements are tied tightly with the balance and detoxification of estrogen.

Finally, a diet low in carbohydrates can also negatively impact a woman's sleep.[32] Nearly all hormones are released according to the circadian rhythm, the natural daily rhythm that both dictates your sleep cycle and is influenced by it. When sleep becomes disrupted because of the keto diet or another factor — a problem more common to women than men — other hormones may become disrupted. Disrupt the rhythm, disrupt the hormones. Not surprisingly, sleep disruption is connected to more visceral fat at the waist.[33]

In the only study of the ketogenic diet suggesting a benefit for women that does not apply to men, female rats on a ketogenic diet didn't lose bone mass, but male rats did.[34] Of course, we need to replicate these data in humans before drawing firm conclusions.

## 5. Women can follow a ketogenic diet, but they do better with a hormone-balancing version such as the Gottfried Protocol.

The primary reasons women don't seem to benefit equally from a ketogenic diet are related to hormones, which can influence effective detoxification, stress and cortisol, thyroid function, hunger and food addiction, and blood sugar levels.

The Gottfried Protocol is a modified keto diet that works better for women. It includes a detox component, a modified carb count, and more vegetables and fiber for a more alkaline diet.[35] In my experience with patients, the Gottfried Protocol contributes to healthy gut function, improved hormones, and significant fat loss. Plus, my patients are not hungry. Finding a plan that works is important, especially when you consider that dietary change could prevent half of all chronic diseases.[36]

Here's an example of how a change in diet affects our health. You see, our bodies have been becoming more acidic since our hunter-gatherer years. Since the agricultural revolution (starting ten thousand years ago) and the industrial revolution (starting two hundred years ago), soils have become increasingly depleted in minerals that we need, such as calcium, magnesium, iron, manganese, copper, and zinc. Standard diets likewise have less magnesium, fiber, and potassium, as compared to sodium; chloride has increased in comparison to bicarbonate. The result is that the food most of us are eating may induce metabolic acidosis: the body's delicate balance between acid and base shifts to the acid side, causing higher blood pressure (see details in the Notes).[37]

All these changes result in a greater risk for kidney stones, which may occur more frequently for people on "lazy keto."[38] Low carb with high protein isn't the right answer; instead, you need to eat more vegetables and other specific foods that boost magnesium, fiber, and potassium. A more alkaline diet that's rich in vegetables will improve hormones like growth hormone, increase levels of vitamin D, help your bones, and reduce muscle loss.[39] That's what you get with the Gottfried Protocol.

I've wondered over the years if the decreased insulin and glucose that we see as a result of the ketogenic diet, or even during fasting, when you go for some period of time without eating (such as fourteen to sixteen hours), might be perceived as a greater alarm in women as compared to men — meaning it sets off warning signals in the female body that something is wrong. I suspect that for women in perimenopause, this alarm might be more sensitive, perhaps requiring gentler methods (like a shorter fasting window of 13 to 14 hours). I have not yet found clear evidence supporting my observations with the ketogenic diet on this point, but fasting for forty-eight hours does seem to trigger a major stress response in overweight premenopausal women (it activates the sympathetic nervous system, producing the fight-flight-freeze response).[40] In contrast, men who do weight lifting (another stressor) experience increased calm, relaxation, reduced blood pressure, and a feeling of being well rested (the parasympathetic activity known as the rest-and-digest response).[41]

Putting it all together, my approach gets my patients pooping and detoxing; adding more carbs, nonstarchy vegetables, and plenty of fiber; and aiming for a more gradual insulin-fixing process, so that we don't shock the female body into a fat-storing panic. You'll get all the details in Part 2.

That's exactly what happened with Melissa. A blood test indicated that she was low in a hormone called DHEA, which is a precursor to testosterone, and low in the mineral magnesium. Her body composition test showed high levels of visceral fat, as reflected in a waist circumference of 39 inches. Other tests showed that she had multiple risk factors for cardiovascular disease, including her cholesterol levels: a rising LDL and a low HDL. She started the Gottfried Protocol — first, we got her pooping, detoxing, and correcting her insulin. Her initial goal was to lose 5 pounds only. Progress with weight loss was slow at first, but steady, and to date she has lost 17 pounds. Even more important, her glucose is now normal and her cholesterol panel is heading in the right direction.

## Is Keto Right for Me?

In this book I will be sharing a well-formulated ketogenic diet, one that is designed with women's issues and hormones in mind. If you have a history of medical conditions (such as gallbladder problems or no gallbladder, cardiovascular disease, or a history of kidney stones), or if you've been told to stay away from high-fat diets, you will want to check with your doctor before starting this diet. You may need additional guidance to try the Gottfried Protocol, such as which specific oils to use if you have gallbladder problems. Absolute and relative contraindications are discussed later in the book, but please ask your clinician for help if you are unsure about any detail.

# *Highlights*

In this chapter, we covered the key precision-medicine principles for women, hormones, and metabolism.

► You learned about how hormones influence weight and which hormones are the most important to know about and to target.

► You discovered that women have more hormone problems than men do, and that over the age of thirty-five and during perimenopause, major changes occur that can make your body resistant to weight loss.

► Women and men differ in terms of how their endocrine system directs fat storage and in their brain responses to signals regulating weight and body fat distribution. You learned that women partition fat more in their subcutaneous space and may become fat in the lower body (hips, butt, thighs — the "pear" shape), whereas men partition fat in their abdomen, in and around their abdominal organs — the "apple" shape. In perimenopause, women may become more like men, with higher insulin levels, lower estrogen levels, weight gain, and fat gain at the waist — hence, more apple-shaped. Polycystic ovary syndrome and insulin resistance can cause the shape too.

► We discussed how the ketogenic diet can address these hormonal changes, but that women react differently to keto. The Gottfried Protocol takes this into account. Specifically, women need to be pooping daily to detoxify and reset their hormones, they need more fiber and nonstarchy vegetables, and they need to pay attention to how carbohydrate restriction might be affecting stress and cortisol levels. You can do the ketogenic diet, but you will react best if you follow the modified version that I cover in Part 2. It will help you optimize your hormones and set yourself up for permanent weight loss.

Fortunately, you can apply the principles of precision medicine to customize your own weight-loss program. In the next few chapters, we will cover a few other hormones in detail, including growth hormone and testosterone, and connect the dots between what you eat and the hormonal symphony.

# 2

## HOW GROWTH HORMONE KEEPS YOU LEAN

When my patient Carrie turned forty-three, she noticed several unwelcome changes. She felt like the normal dewiness of her skin and volume of her muscle had changed, and she showed me photographic evidence on her smartphone. Throughout her life, she felt generally calm and collected; now she had bouts of anxiety. Her energy was lower. It was harder to recover from a night of poor sleep or a workout. Looking in the mirror, she saw more sagging skin and less muscle. Even more frustrating, she'd gained stubborn extra pounds since having kids, mostly concentrated at her waist, but none of her usual diet tactics were working. Determined to get to her goal weight of 130 pounds, she explained that a typical day followed a standard "mom" diet formula: oatmeal with fruit for breakfast, multiple cans of diet soda, a small salad at lunch, and a take-out dinner, washed down with a few glasses of wine. Low calorie — well, except for all that wine.

I asked about her sleep, and she confessed that she was going to bed later than she used to, more like 11 p.m. or midnight, after streaming video with her partner, and her sleep was not as solid. When I examined Carrie, I noticed saggy cheeks and thin lips. I agreed that overall she didn't have much muscle tone, considering her age and how much she worked out at the gym.

Perhaps you can relate to Carrie's struggles. You may even think that her complaints are the unavoidable results of aging, but I disagree. I suspected that hormones were to blame for her recent weight gain, her challenge with the scale, her frustrating drop in energy, and her body's general lack of definition. In fact, a hormonal switch was to blame — that is, the toggle between "let's burn fat" and "let's store fat," controlled in her body by several key hormones.

Carrie was surprised to hear that her daily food choices weren't helping her lose weight because they were activating the wrong hormones. At first my concern about a faulty hormonal switch barely registered with her. Then a simple blood test confirmed that I was right, which meant that Carrie's "mom" diet was effective at packing on more pounds, not helping them come off, and it was exacerbating her hormone imbalance. Let me explain.

## HORMONES:
## THE MISSING KEY

A hormone is a substance that regulates function in the body. It is produced in the body and transported in fluids such as the blood in order to tell a distant cell what to do. Hormones can be inside the body (endogenous) or made in a lab from animals or plants and given to someone (exogenous), in over-the-counter form or by prescription. Hormones influence behavior, mood, muscle mass, energy, and metabolism. They drive what you are interested in and want to focus on, like eating or burning fat or having sex. Often, hormones are cited to disparage or dismiss women, as in *"You're hormonal! Get it together!"* In reality, hormones influence our behavior, and our behavior can influence our hormones. First, let's see how hormones work and then what we can do about them.

## Hormones That Influence the Body's Fat Management

Three hormones play a key role in the hormonal switch that can take you from storing fat to burning fat.

**Growth hormone** stimulates growth and cell regeneration. As a kid, it makes you taller. As an adult, it keeps your muscles lean by building muscle and burning fat. Unfortunately, growth hormone declines slowly as you age, beginning around age thirty, especially if you experience a lot of stress, eat carbs throughout the day, sit too much, and don't exercise enough.

**Testosterone** is the most abundant hormone in both men and women, and it plays a central role in functions similar to those of growth hormone, including building muscle and burning fat. Testosterone is now recognized as a multitasking hormone in women, involved in keeping metabolism strong and libido healthy. Like growth hormone, it declines in your thirties but drops more precipitously in perimenopause and menopause.

**Insulin** regulates the amount of glucose in your blood. In healthy folks, when the pancreas detects that too much glucose is in the bloodstream, insulin signals muscles, the liver, and other tissues to absorb it and convert it to energy. If you eat excess carbohydrates or don't manage stress well, insulin becomes blocked and glucose rises in the blood, and at high levels it can be toxic. This is called insulin resistance: your cells become numb to the insulin message. This condition is a precursor to diabetes (prediabetes) and can lead to greater hunger and more fat storage, particularly at the belly.

Growth hormone is a build-you-up hormone, meaning that it plays a key role in building muscle and keeping bones strong, while simultaneously breaking down fat. It's central to weight loss, and problems with growth hormone may be less recognized in women compared to men. Growth hormone made you became taller as a child. For adults, growth hormone is still involved in growth and repair, including bone mineralization, protein synthesis, cellular growth, and fat breakdown. We have naturally lower levels of growth hormone as we age. Production peaks in early adulthood but then declines by 1 to 3 percent per year after age thirty — a decline that's much more precipitous than that of other hormones, and therefore may be more noticeable.[1] Many of my female patients notice the telltale signs of a fat, droopy abdomen and loss of muscle tone. One thirty-seven-year-old patient with low growth hormone calls it the "melted candle" look.

It's relatively easy to test your growth hormone levels. To confirm my suspicion of Carrie's low growth hormone, we ordered a blood test that's a proxy for growth hormone, called IGF-1, and we found she was, indeed, low. (IGF-1 is a growth factor produced by the liver when stimulated by a rise in growth hormone. IGF-1 is easier to measure than growth hormone.)

Testosterone functions overlap with growth hormone in that it builds muscle and boosts metabolism. Both growth hormone and testosterone are multitasking hormones, performing more than one job in the body. For example, testosterone can boost your mood and sense of confidence while helping you build muscle in the gym, and it helps your thyroid work better. (You will learn more about testosterone and how to activate it for weight loss in the next chapter.)

## BOOSTING GROWTH HORMONE

You might wonder if you can just take a pill to boost your growth hormone and watch the pounds melt off your middle. Unfortunately, no. But when we look at the factors that determine your growth hormone — age, sex, diet, nutrition, food timing, sleep, and exercise — you'll soon realize that many of these are within your power to manipulate to your advantage.

The goal with the Gottfried Protocol is to get your hormones, including the essential growth hormone, back into balance. You don't want growth hormone to dip too low, or you may feel prematurely old, like Carrie. You may feel frail before your time, and even note a loss of brain power.[2] But you also don't want to crank growth hormone up too high as it may be associated with a greater risk of cancer. You want it to be in balance, and eating the right food, in the right quantities, and at the right time are the most important drivers.

## Growth Hormone Questionnaire

Do you have or have you experienced any of the following symptoms in the past six months?

- Do you notice signs of premature aging, such as a sagging face, thin lips, droopy eyelids, or wrinkles?
- Do you feel less inner peace or calm than in the past? *Y* Have you experienced more anxious feelings that lack a specific cause?
- Is your height normal, but you're beginning to hunch over? *N*
- Examine your hands. Do you notice thinning muscles, such as reduced muscle tone at the palm of the hands, especially just beneath the thumb and under the little finger? *Y*
- When you pinch the skin at the back of the hand for 3 seconds, does your skin immediately snap back, or is it delayed? (This is also a test for dehydration.) *snap back*
- Look at your nails. Do you see striae, or longitudinal lines?
- Do you have increased stretch marks on the abdomen? *N*
- Do you have more belly fat than in the past, especially at your waistline? *Y*
- Are your inner thighs saggy? *Y*
- Do you have fatty cushions (fat deposits) above the knees? *Y*

- Are you experiencing more difficulty in performing common daily tasks?
- Are you noticing a change in emotional reactions? Are you more reactive than you used to be, giving sharp verbal retorts to comments that may not have bothered you in the past?
- Do you feel colder than others while at the same ambient temperature? Do you need to wear socks to bed? (In medicine, we refer to this issue as cold intolerance.)
- Are you noticing that your muscles are less pronounced than they used to be? When you exercise regularly, do you notice less of a muscle response or a loss of strength? *y*
- Have you been diagnosed with osteopenia (less bone density compared to your peers) or osteoporosis? Have *N* you been diagnosed with a fracture?
- Have you noticed diffuse thinning of body hair?
- Are you noticing that your quality of life has declined? *y*
- Is your sleep light or disrupted? Are you going to bed *y* later than usual? (The first three to four hours of sleep each night are the time when you produce the highest levels of growth hormone.)

*Please note: If you are experiencing excessive worry that interferes with relationships, work, or other aspects of your life, it's time to talk to a licensed mental health professional or doctor about whether you have an anxiety disorder.*

### Interpreting Your Results

If you answered yes to five or more of the questions above, you may have low growth hormone. Don't panic — it's easy to reverse low growth hormone if you get help sooner rather than later. Read on to learn more about low growth hormone, its root cause, and how the Gottfried Protocol can help.

# THE SCIENCE OF
# LOW GROWTH HORMONE

If science makes you run for the hills, here's the short version of what depletes growth hormone: *lack of sleep, lack of exercise, tons of stress,* and *munching on carbs all day long.* Hmmm, sounds like my thirties. Now, you may still be in denial and think to yourself, "No, not me," but let's take a deeper look. Mothering two kids led to profound sleep deprivation for me and probably bottomed out my growth hormone. When I went back to work after having each kid, I was basically sedentary and running on stress (that is, high cortisol). Who had time for the luxury of exercise? I felt almost constantly hypoglycemic, so each day was a blur of many things that cranked up my blood sugar: fruit, energy bars, and chips.

Growth hormone is a crucial hormone that—among its numerous roles—keeps you lean and energized. When everything is in check, growth hormone works harmoniously with your hormones cortisol and adrenaline to burn fat and build muscle. As mentioned earlier, growth hormone is a component of the hormonal switch between burning glucose to burning fat.[3] We'll be discussing this hormonal switch in greater detail in this chapter and the next few, as we cover the jobs of three hormones: growth hormone, testosterone, and insulin. For now, it's important to know that sometimes the switch gets stuck in the "store fat" position because the body perceives too much stress due to deadlines, restricted calories or other famine signals, overexercise, insufficient sleep, or toxins.

High levels of growth hormone, as measured by blood levels of IGF-1, are associated with better cognitive function.[4] Most people think that hormones like growth hormone gradually decline with age, and that's true to a certain extent. But I've found that the drop is more precipitous in my female patients who struggle with their weight and have loads of stress. In fact, the level of growth hormone that you had when you were an adolescent (that's ages ten to nineteen, according to the World Health Organization) was *eight hundred times* the level of other hormones, such as the one that regulates thyroid hormone production or the hormone that helps control ovulation.[5] (I know, *eight hundred* seems like a typo—it's not!) I imagine that because production is so high and then drops so exponentially, during early middle age it can hit some of us especially hard.

You may wonder why you should care about growth hormone. Here's the skinny. **When growth hormone (and other hormonal) levels are optimal, you can enjoy benefits including fat loss or easy weight maintenance, increased energy and stamina, and more.** Trouble starts when hormones become unruly or your body stops making sufficient growth hormone. Studies show that impaired levels can increase fat, break down muscle, decrease energy[6]—and generally make life miserable. Low growth hormone is even one of the markers for frailty as you age.[7] Here are some other symptoms of growth hormone deficiency:

- Reduced lean body mass
- Increased abdominal obesity
- Increased insulin resistance, leading to prediabetes and type 2 diabetes
- Decreased muscle mass
- Hypertension (high blood pressure)
- High triglycerides (high levels of a type of fat in the blood)
- Anxiety and depression
- Fibromyalgia
- Decreased bone density

## GROWTH HORMONE IN WOMEN

Women make growth hormone differently than men do. Before menopause, women tend to have higher levels of it.[8] As is the case for a few other hormones, you don't make it continuously, but rather you produce growth hormone in pulses—and mostly at night, while you sleep. Men have longer periods of time between pulses of growth hormone; women produce it more continuously, with only short intervals between those pulses.[9] IGF-1 levels are lower in women compared to men after age fifty — perhaps this is because women are more than twice as likely to suffer from insomnia.[10] Another difference is related to exercise. When men and women engage in anaerobic exercise (intense, shorter exercise, such as burpees, box jumps, and sprints, which break down glucose without oxygen), women produce higher levels of growth hormone as a result.[11] And peak production occurs twice as soon in women (20 minutes after exercise) compared to men (40 minutes after exercise). We can use that to our advantage to boost growth hormone and lose fat!

If growth hormone is such a good thing, and we all make less as we age,[12] why do some people experience a more dramatic drop than others? Besides the factors already mentioned (eating too much sugar, not exercising enough, experiencing a great deal of stress, and so forth), too much belly fat and a decline in sex hormones (examples: estrogen, testosterone) can contribute to the drop.

Though you cannot control your chronological age, you can control belly fat. Abdominal fat plays more of a factor in growth hormone decline than age does, according to one study in the *Journal of Clinical Endocrinology and Metabolism*. This is true even for people who are not obese.[13]

## GROWTH HORMONE AFFECTS OTHER HORMONES TOO

Growth hormone, cortisol, and insulin are interconnected, and when they go haywire, problems ensue. For instance, one study found that overweight adolescent girls with high cortisol and low growth hormone stored more belly fat and had increased insulin resistance,[14] setting the stage for obesity and diabetes. Combine stress, poor sleep, and inadequate growth hormone levels with a diet high in sugar and processed foods, and you've got a formula for feeling lousy, lethargic, and out of juice. Here are the other hormone imbalances that may impact growth hormone and contribute to metabolic inflexibility.

- **Insulin block.** In this condition, insulin is no longer able to push glucose efficiently inside a cell, and the cell becomes numb to the effects of insulin; this is common in children and adults with growth hormone deficiency.[15]
- **Leptin.** Adults who lack growth hormone have higher levels of leptin, the hormone that tells you to stop eating. These higher levels indicate leptin block, and folks who experience this often feel hungry all the time.[16]
- **Estrogen.** As women age and estrogen declines, growth hormone declines.[17] Estrogen, among its many other jobs, suppresses appetite. That's why women over forty often need a new strategy to get growth hormone in balance.
- **Testosterone.** Adults who are low in growth hormone make less DHEA, the hormone that is the precursor (building block) to testosterone.[18] (Chapter 3 will cover the androgen family, including DHEA and testosterone.)
- **Others.** Additional hormones that influence growth hormone are mentioned in the Notes, including but not limited to thyroid hormone, luteinizing hormone, and follicle stimulating hormone.[19]

## MEET MOLLY

Molly was a forty-nine-year-old patient who came to my precision medicine practice because her mood felt flat, sort of "blah" and muted, and her body felt pudgy. Normally she was a high-energy, life-of-the-party type, so this was new for her. Her internist, after administering a single thyroid test (thyroid stimulating hormone or TSH, the typical screening test for low thyroid function), told her she was just getting older. More extensive testing revealed several hormone issues: not only was her IGF-1 low, indicating low growth hormone, but her thyroid function was borderline slow (as measured by multiple tests, covered in the Notes).[20] Her levels of testosterone and estrogen had decreased but were "normal" for menopause, and her fasting insulin was creeping up. With my guidance, Molly began a new food plan that included morning whey protein shakes, detoxification, and intermittent fasting. I initiated a low dose of thyroid medication. Within eight weeks, her IGF-1 was up by 32 percent, she had gained 2 pounds of muscle, she had lost 12 pounds of fat, and best of all, her energy was back.

## HOW TO FIX THE GROWTH HORMONE DEFICIT

Let's correct your whispering growth hormone and muscle loss. Here is my prescription for what to do. You'll find recipes, meal plans, and the support you need in Part 2.

- **Eat healthy protein.** You can raise IGF-1 by eating protein, particularly proteins rich in the amino acid called methionine. The goal is balance; you want to get the right amount of protein for you — not too much and not too little. However, many of the studies of protein consumption are limited to men. According to one, for men of ages forty to seventy-five, both animal and vegetable proteins raise IGF-1;[21] in a smaller study of men, only red meat increased it.[22] In women, higher protein intake has been associated with higher levels of IGF-1, but the association was limited to animal protein and did not apply to vegetable protein.[23] Other research in athletes shows that whey protein shakes are particularly helpful at raising IGF-1 and testosterone,[24] boosting IGF-1 in postmenopausal women,[25] and increasing muscle mass in older folks.[26] Think foods like grass-fed, grass-finished beef (from pasture-fed cows never fattened with grain, which increases inflammation); SMASH fish (salmon, mackerel, anchovies, sardines, and herring); whey protein shakes; and pastured eggs and chicken. Carrie drank a whey protein shake every morning during her workout (about 10 minutes into weight lifting) and added SMASH fish most days of the week. For dinner, she alternated poached eggs with grass-fed, grass-finished beef twice per week.

- **Eat healthy fats.** Omega-3s have been shown to raise growth hormone in animal studies.[27] If you have increased belly fat and insulin and blood sugar problems — a common driver of weight gain, inflammation, and even breast cancer — your body may be producing more of the type of fats that make you inflamed and resistant to weight loss.[28] Consuming a healthy mix of omega fats can help your body be more sensitive to insulin and keep the fat-burning switch in the "on" position. Not surprisingly, eating more omega-3s as found in flaxseed and SMASH fish, which creates a higher ratio of omega-3s to omega-6s, has been shown to reduce breast cancer by 27 percent.[29] Add medium-chain triglyceride (MCT) oil and chia seeds to your smoothie, and macadamia nuts and avocado oil to your salad. Top it off with a square of dark chocolate. I provide more information on what and how much to eat in Part 2.

- **Fast.** You may have heard about the fasting diet trend. Multiple studies show that intermittent fasting increases growth hormone.[30] An animal experiment suggested that fasting is more likely to stimulate the fat-burning benefit of growth hormone,[31] which is why a 14/10 protocol (fourteen hours of overnight fasting, and ten hours for your eating window — for instance, stop eating by 6 p.m. and then eat breakfast at 8 a.m. each day) is part of the Gottfried Protocol. One study found a twenty-four-hour fasting period boosted growth hormone at an average of 1,300 percent in women and almost 2,000 percent in men.[32] It's not fair — I know! But research shows there is a benefit to fasting for both men and women, even if men see a greater increase in growth hormone.

- **Exercise.** Exercise raises growth hormone and IGF-1, and the more strenuous, the greater the effect.[33] Personally, I raised my IGF-1 by 53 percent over eight weeks with high-intensity interval training. I became interested in exercise as a way to boost IGF-1 when a friend taught me about high-intensity interval training, using a method of maximal effort for 60 to 75 seconds followed by 1 to 2 minutes of rest, for a total of eight rounds. (See "Raising IGF-1 with Exercise" on page 56 for details.) IGF-1 mediates many of the beneficial effects of exercise on brain health and function.

- **Take a sauna.**[34] Sauna bathing for 30 to 60 minutes raises growth hormone up to 140 percent after a single session.[35]
- **Put down the wine (and other alcoholic beverages).** If your growth hormone is out of balance, alcohol may lower it further.[36] While on the Gottfried Protocol, abstain from drinking. Think of alcohol as liquid sugar — it goes directly to the liver and can be converted into fat. Unless you're at your goal weight and body fat, avoid alcohol. It will clog your liver, hinder detoxification, and make you puffy and resistant to weight loss.
- **Consider supplements.** Some key supplements can help increase growth hormone; they include vitamin D (aim for serum vitamin D level 60 to 90 ng/mL) and creatine (15–20 g/d for five days, thereafter 3–5 g/d), which have been shown to help men and women with declining muscle mass.[37] Vitamin D is a hormone that has over four hundred jobs in the body and has been shown in twenty-five randomized trials to reduce risk of viral infection.[38]
- **Can I just get a growth hormone shot?** You may wonder why you can't just take a growth hormone prescription and top off your low levels. Unfortunately, long-term studies of growth hormone administration show conflicting safety results, so the Food and Drug Administration has very strict guidelines. In a nutshell, injecting yourself with growth hormone is not something I recommend due to side effects, including joint pain, swelling, carpal tunnel syndrome,[39] and cancer, particularly of the breast, colon, and prostate.[40] As you will learn in Chapter 6, if weight loss is still elusive on the Gottfried Protocol, you may want to discuss with your physician a prescription for peptides that help boost growth hormone, known as growth hormone *secretagogues*.[41]

## Raising IGF-1 with Exercise

When I was forty-six, I used exercise to raise my blood level of IGF-1 from 219 to 334 ng/mL in an N-of-1 experiment. It wasn't a huge commitment; it was 20 minutes, four days per week, to be exact. Let me explain.

I've been exercising for years. Not because I love it but because I need it for my brain and weight. I heard from a friend about something called "Sprint 8" and decided to try it. Sprint 8 is a system for high-intensity interval training (HIIT) that's super-efficient, with eight rounds of burst training interspersed with recovery at your usual moderate level of exercise.

Here's how I did it. I didn't perform any other exercise, just Sprint 8 four times per week.

- Jog at moderate pace for 3 to 5 minutes. I have a genetic tendency toward an Achilles injury, so I warm up for 5 to 10 minutes first and always stretch my Achilles. For me, a moderate jogging pace is a 12-minute mile, or 5 miles per hour on a treadmill.
- Sprint all out for 30 seconds, so hard you can't go more than 30 seconds.
- Recover for 75 to 90 seconds. If you have trouble with math or have more time to spare, I encourage going for 90 seconds.
- Lather, rinse, repeat. Repeat the sprint for a total of eight cycles.
- Cool down at your moderate pace.

After six weeks, I retested my IGF-1 and it had risen to 334, an increase of 53 percent. My weight was about the same, but at the time, I didn't have weight to lose. My body fat was lower. My waist circumference decreased. *It worked!*

Carrie raised her IGF-1 by 40 percent over four weeks by following the Gottfried Protocol and consequently lost 15 pounds, including 12 pounds of fat. In the next chapter, you'll learn more about testosterone, a close cousin of growth hormone with overlapping functions — and another metabolic hormone you can activate to lose fat more easily.

## *Highlights*

Growth hormone is one of the top metabolic hormones with a prominent role in weight, health, and fitness.[42]

- ▶ Keeping growth hormone balanced helps maintain your body fat, lean muscle mass, bone, tendons, and brain function. It also builds your brain, skin, hair, internal organs, and bones.
- ▶ Having too much growth hormone is associated with cancer risk, which is why you want to use diet and other targeted lifestyle interventions to keep this hormone in balance rather than taking a prescription shot.
- ▶ The key with growth hormone is balance — you don't want too little, and you don't want too much.

# 3

## TESTOSTERONE:
### It's Not Just for Men

Nicole made a telehealth appointment because, at age forty-four, she was experiencing middle-age spread. She pointed to her flabby muscles — and no amount of time in the gym seemed to help. She grabbed a fistful of what she considered to be too round of a belly, and then pointed to her back fat, or "hate handles," as she called them. The increased belly and back fat were new.

I am careful to normalize body fat. We need it to make hormones, and we need healthy fat in our diet to build hormones. Having cholesterol levels that are not too high and not too low drive hormonal, mental, and physical health. Eating healthy fat does not make us fat. On the other hand, visceral fat is part of that worsening continuum from metabolic flexibility to inflexibility that I mentioned — that's why I measure it in all of my patients.

When I asked about her mood, she confided that she felt more fearful about her future, less assertive at work. She told me about other woes: night sweats, hemorrhoids, sciatica, a recent bone screening showing osteopenia (age-related bone loss), not cooking at home as much and eating cereal for dinner, less interest in physical activity. When we got to her sexual history, I asked about sex drive. Nicole shifted uncomfortably in her seat and replied: "Near zero." Finally, I asked about her values and how that related to the reason she made her appointment. She told me she wants to be healthier, add more years to her life, and experience more of the wonderful things life has to offer.

We measured her waist at 36 inches, and weight at 144 pounds (at 5 feet 2 inches tall, her body mass index or BMI was in the overweight range at 26.3, and her body fat was in the obese range at 33 percent). Her hormones were sputtering in perimenopause. When we ran a few blood tests, most striking were her low testosterone and DHEA levels. I knew exactly what to do to help her.

You likely know testosterone (known as "T" for short) as the *male* sex hormone. But women make T too. We don't have testes like men do, so we make it in our ovaries, as well as in cells within the adrenal glands, fat, skin, and brain.[1] Overall, healthy men have ten to twenty times the levels of healthy women, but while men have more, T is the *most abundant biologically active hormone* in women. Yes, T is more abundant in the female body than even estrogen. You have receptors for T throughout your body, from the brain to the breast to the vagina and many places in between. In fact, given women's lower level of T compared to men's, you might even say that women are exquisitely sensitive to it.

Most women have plenty of T — and its precursor, DHEA (see the box on page 64) — until their twenties, when their levels begin to decline.[2] That's one reason why young women typically have a lot of energy, sex drive, and confidence, as well as muscle and bone strength, and don't have as hard a time keeping their weight in the normal range. T is a build-you-up hormone, like growth hormone, meaning that it aids in the construction of the body — from bones to muscles to skin — and simultaneously breaks down fat. But T has an even broader job description. While it's involved in body composition and muscle mass, it also plays a central role in sex drive, mood, and well-being. Women require adequate levels to feel vital and lean, cell to soul.

That's why, as women age and their T plummets, many of them experience a reduction in energy, sex drive, strength, the ability to maintain a healthy weight, and that basic feeling of health and vitality. My clinical experience confirms this: In my patients, women at age forty have half the level of T of women in their twenties, and many of them have complaints like Nicole's.

To determine if your T levels may be low, fill out the following questionnaire.

## Testosterone Questionnaire

Do you have or have you experienced any of the following symptoms in the past six months?

- Do you have a normal female pattern of body hair, but the hair is thinning – particularly under your arms and in the pubic area?
- Do you notice signs of premature hair loss on the head, at the temples (sides of the forehead)?
- Do you like physical activity and sports, but your interest has been fading recently?
- Have you experienced intense emotional stress or trauma as an adult?
- Are you a long-distance runner or do you engage in other regular endurance exercise?
- Has your sex drive declined gradually since your twenties?
- Is your clitoris less sensitive than it used to be, which makes stimulation to orgasm take longer or require more effort?
- Is vaginal intercourse painful or irritating?
- Do you feel more passive, or less likely to take risks in daily life?
- Do you feel more fragile and excessively sensitive

to difficulties, as if your resistance to stress is diminished? 4
- Do you feel depressive or tend to cling to a negative point of view? Y
- Are your muscles reduced in volume, tone, and strength?
- Have you noticed more cellulite and/or varicose veins?
- Is your skin thin, dry, and/or easily sunburned?
- Are you experiencing more joint pain, particularly low back pain?
- Do you have dry eyes?
- Have you lost height? Become more hunched over with your posture? N
- Is your body scent diminished?
- Do you have fat accumulation at the breasts, waist, and/or hips? Y

If you answered yes to five or more of the questions above, you may have low T, and I recommend you proceed as if you do. You can raise low T with lifestyle changes like diet and exercise if you get help early. If you wait until too late, the only option may be to discuss T replacement with a trusted and well-educated clinician who can discuss the risks and benefits. If you are uncertain or want additional confirmation, consider getting tested for T, through a blood or urine test. Suggested labs are mentioned in the Notes, which are commonly ordered by most conventional gynecologists.[3]

## LOW T IN WOMEN

While low T is a well-recognized problem in men, the implications of T deficiency — and the benefits of T therapy — in women have long been the subject of debate. Many doctors don't think about T when female patients complain of low energy, low sex drive, flab (as in Nicole's case), weight gain, or an inability to lose weight in the ways that used to work when they were younger. There are many other surprising symptoms of low T in women, from bonier hands to a less sensitive clitoris (see the questionnaire for a more complete list), which can be uncomfortable, embarrassing, inconvenient, or just depressing, and they can begin to surface in women as early as their midthirties.

So why are doctors so oblivious at best, or dismissive at worst, concerning low T in women? Why do many of them fail to test for it? A dearth of publicized research means that many physicians have no idea that levels decline steeply during a woman's reproductive years, especially for those who undergo removal of their ovaries (called oophorectomy, this is sometimes performed along with a hysterectomy to treat or prevent ovarian cancer).[4] Also, most physicians don't recognize the benefits of identifying and treating women who are suffering with low T. But even if doctors think of low T as a possible problem, test for it, and want to treat it, there are currently no FDA-approved treatments for low T in women. They have to wing it, or prescribe something off-label, or prescribe something that hasn't been well tested in women, and that can be something a lot of doctors hesitate to do.

While you may not get the kind of response you would like from your doctor, and while controversy continues to exist regarding T therapy for women who are deficient, fortunately, there are solutions available for you. Therapeutic lifestyle intervention — especially dietary factors — can help significantly boost your levels of androgens (the so-called male hormones, including T and its precursor, DHEA) when you are low.

## In the Androgens Family, Testosterone Is the Star

T is one type of androgen. Androgens are so-called "male" hormones (*andro-* is a Greek term for "man") that are present in higher concentrations in men than women. They are responsible for male sexual development, sperm count, and sex drive, as well as secondary sexual characteristics like muscle and bone growth, facial and body hair growth, and a deep voice. They can also influence energy and mood.

The other androgens besides T include androstenedione, dihydrotestosterone (DHT), dehydroepiandrosterone (DHEA), and dehydroepiandrosterone sulfate (DHEA-S). Each of these is complexly related to different actions in the body. For example, DHT is linked to balding, and DHEA is a hormone that is used to make both T and estrogen and is also related to immunity, mood, cognition, strength, and aging (or *not* aging — it is sometimes called the "anti-aging hormone"). DHEA-S is involved in the onset of puberty in youth and in stress throughout life; also, it can be a factor in the onset of dementia in old age.

Just as men have a lot of androgens and some (but a much smaller amount) estrogens, women have a lot of estrogens and a much smaller amount of androgens. (As mentioned, we still have more T in total amount than estrogens.) Both sexes need both types of sex hormones. When women experience decreasing levels of androgens with age, they tend to experience reduced sex drive, feel more tired, and just don't feel as well as they once did, even if they can't pinpoint specific symptoms. (In men, since T is used to create the estrogen called estradiol, decreased T often leads to decreased estrogen, which is linked to increased body fat and weaker muscles.)

# THE SCIENCE OF
# LOW TESTOSTERONE
# IN WOMEN

There are a number of reasons why low T is common in women. For one thing, your body naturally makes less T as you get older, but natural menopause has less of an effect on T levels than you might think — the drop in T typically precedes menopause by many years. There is a dramatic 50 percent reduction between ages twenty and forty, and DHEA drops even more precipitously than T as you age.[5] The exception is surgical menopause — when your ovaries are removed, T plummets.[6] Otherwise, the loss of T is gradual and not dramatic with menopause. Another potential cause of low T: the birth control pill. It raises sex hormone binding globulin (SHBG), which is like a sponge that carries T around the body and tends to lower your free T levels.[7]

While lower T can be a natural thing, what I've found in my practice to be one of the biggest contributors to unnaturally low levels of T in women is lifestyle — especially diet.

Another common reason for low T is a medication: statins for high cholesterol. Not only that, but statins deplete many phytonutrients (see the list in Notes).[8] The television ads suggest statins are a panacea, but the truth is that they are a very common cause of declining T, and even a severe form of muscle breakdown called rhabdomyolysis. Most of the research has focused on men, but the effect applies to women as well.[9]

Why you have low T can help you determine your solution, but similar to the research on growth hormone, much of the research on raising T with diet and other lifestyle factors comes from studies on men. Still, we can take much of what we already know about how to increase T and apply it to *you*. I've done this with my patients and seen great results.

# WHY TESTOSTERONE IS
# IMPORTANT FOR WOMEN

I've already hinted at why you want and need T, but let's look more closely at what else it can do for you.

If you're trying to get leaner and lose more body fat, T is an important ally. It is the hormone that creates a weight-loss edge for men. It generally helps men build more muscle mass and gives them a higher resting metabolic rate — that is, men tend to burn more calories at rest than women do. Since women produce less T than men, we have less muscle mass and a lower metabolic rate — which is why men lose weight and gain muscle more easily than women do. I suspect this is why the ketogenic diet, which involves higher fat, moderate protein, and low carbohydrate intake, tends to work better for men, according to my research. The Gottfried Protocol follows a ketogenic framework but is adapted for women, together with detoxification and fasting.

Wishing you were in the mood more often? T and the other androgens are the main hormones that fuel sex drive in both men and women, and T levels are positively linked with the ability to have an orgasm.[10] Women with low DHEA have a higher likelihood of low sexual desire at all ages from eighteen to seventy-five (though some with low DHEA have a normal sex drive).[11] According to other studies, the free level of T — or "free" T, meaning, the amount that is biologically available to bind to receptors, the way a lock fits into a key — matters more than total T, which is calculated as free T plus the amount of T bound to carriers in the blood.[12] Of course, T isn't the only factor in a healthy libido. For women, context is also very important — that includes relationship satisfaction, emotional support, self-esteem, optimism, the presence of pain, contentment, and life satisfaction.[13] However, there is no denying that T and other androgens play a role in translating those emotional elements into a physical response.

Not feeling so cheerful lately? T may also be involved in mood and cognition, though data on this possibility are more limited.[14]

DHEA (that precursor to T) may also be a remedy for severe stress, as measured by cortisol levels. The way DHEA supplements seem to reduce the effects of the stress response after severe trauma may mean it could be a therapy to reduce risk of post-traumatic health problems and even death.[15]

If fertility is a concern, you may be interested to hear that DHEA and T are being explored in assisted reproduction, especially for women with aging eggs.[16] That's an area of research to keep an eye on.

Feeling sluggish and wondering if your thyroid is to blame? Androgens to the rescue yet again. Healthy T levels help regulate the conversion of inactive thyroid hormone (T4) to active thyroid hormone (T3), which can increase thyroid hormone levels that so often decline as women age, but that are also too low in many younger women, for a variety of reasons. A thyroid hormone boost can help you reenergize, so that you can again experience that light and springy feeling.

Maybe you, like Nicole, just want to get healthier in general. Studies show that impaired T levels are associated with several serious health conditions that involve the immune system, inflammation, and glucose problems, including depression, breast cancer, obesity, type 2 diabetes, and Alzheimer's disease.[17]

In the breast, as an example, T may decrease the abnormal growth of cells and density of the breast on a mammogram, but if too much T is converted to estrogen, the risk of breast cancer may rise.[18] For mood, women with low T may benefit from topping off their T with a prescription.[19] It's a case of delicate balance.

## TOO MUCH T

As you can see, T is a boon to women's health in multiple significant ways. However, too much of a good thing is not such a good thing, and with androgens, more is not necessarily better. As with all hormones, balance is everything. Excess T in women is a top reason for infertility, irregular periods, and cardiovascular disease. It could also contribute indirectly to breast cancer risk. T, as you may recall, is converted from DHEA, and then converted to a type of estrogen called estradiol.[20] Too much of this specific type of estrogen could put you at greater risk for breast cancer. Ideally, you want a healthy balance between protective androgens like T (and its precursor DHEA), which may reduce your risk of breast cancer, and stimulatory estrogens like estradiol, which may raise your risk of breast cancer.

Too much T also raises your risk of diabetes and obesity, as can occur with polycystic ovary syndrome (PCOS), a condition in which T levels are abnormally high. PCOS is a complex condition that may be difficult to diagnose, but most women who have it share certain metabolic and mental health symptoms. (See Notes for additional information.)[21] Up to 75 percent of women with PCOS are overweight. While losing weight is hard enough for most people, women with PCOS have an even harder time, probably because of their high insulin levels, which trigger the body to hoard fat. High insulin increases hunger and carbohydrate cravings, making a tough situation even more difficult.

When you have too much T circulating in your bloodstream (as with PCOS), it can stimulate your hair follicles to thicken and grow, resulting in increased growth of body and facial hair. Hirsutism, or excess hair growth, in a male pattern, is present in 80 percent of women with excess androgens. Another marker that's important in dealing with PCOS is a deficiency of SHBG (the sponge that soaks up free T). Women with PCOS who have low levels of SHBG are at greater risk of the metabolic issues I just mentioned, such as blood sugar imbalances.[22]

What helps with PCOS from a dietary perspective? Low-carb[23] and ketogenic diets,[24] which may help to rebalance T when it's too high.

Again, balance is the key. When T (and other hormone) levels are optimally balanced, you can enjoy benefits like fat loss, increased energy and stamina, higher libido, easier orgasms, lower disease risk, more confidence, and a buoyant mood.

The goal with the Gottfried Protocol is to get your hormones back into balance, and that includes T. You want the right amount — not too little, and not too much. If T drops too low, you may feel apathetic and flabby. But you also don't want T to climb too high, as that can put you at risk for conditions like PCOS.

## WHAT YOU CAN DO ABOUT LOW TESTOSTERONE

In order to boost low T levels, the first and most important step you can take is to *improve your diet* — and not just generally, but in some very specific ways. First, let's look at the foods that science has linked with low T in men. In my experience, these foods likely have the same effect in women. You will notice that the lists below are in line with ketogenic principles — cut the carbohydrates, consume moderate protein, and get healthy fats in your diet. The foods associated with lower T are as follows:

- Bread, both refined and whole grain.
- Pastries, and all similar foods made with flour.
- Sugar-sweetened beverages. Consumption of sugar-packed drinks is significantly associated with low serum T in men of ages twenty to thirty-nine in the United States.[25] A single serving of a sugar and protein drink lowers T by 19 percent in overweight and obese boys,[26] and a single oral glucose load drops T by 25 percent in men.[27]
- Coffee. Both caffeinated and decaffeinated coffee decrease T in a randomized trial involving women; men, by contrast, experienced a rise in T after drinking caffeinated coffee.[28] A study in premenopausal women confirmed these results,[29] while a separate study in postmenopausal women showed that drinking caffeine as coffee or other caffeinated beverages is associated with lower bioavailable T.[30] However, data from an observational study are contradictory, showing potential benefits and drawbacks to caffeine.[31] (Randomized trials are less likely to be biased, and they are considered a higher level of evidence compared to observational studies.)
- Diet beverages.

- Dairy products (milk, yogurt, cheese, ice cream, and so forth).
- Desserts in general (in other words, foods with a lot of sugar).
- Restaurant food.[32]

Now let's look at foods and behaviors associated with higher T, more muscle mass, and less visceral fat:

- Homemade food. Make your kitchen the best restaurant around.
- Dark-green vegetables.
- Sufficient but not excess protein (about 0.75 to 1.0 grams per pound of lean body mass—less if you are sedentary and more if you are very active with exercise).
- Exercise, for men. Keto has been shown to raise T in men who exercise.[33]
- Certain herbs, including fenugreek, tribulus, and ginkgo biloba dry extracts, shown to improve T levels. These herbs have been studied in combination to help boost low sex drive among women.[34] Studies suggest that fenugreek[35] and tribulus[36] may be helpful when taken individually as well. These herbs are available at your local health food store.
- Detoxification and removal of endocrine disruptors.

## How Much Protein Do You Need?

I'm a fan of moderate protein intake because excess protein gets converted into sugar in the body, driving up your insulin, driving down your T, and potentially making you store more fat. Moderate protein means 3 to 4 ounces of wild-caught fish. Two eggs, a few times per week. One ounce of nuts or seeds. (For more details, see Chapter 5.) For instance, a woman weighing 130 pounds, with 100 pounds of lean body mass, should eat about 85 to 100 grams of protein each day, or enough to preserve lean body mass. Athletes may need more protein to maintain or increase muscle mass.

## Bisphenol A and Testosterone

One of the worst culprits when it comes to blocking T is the androgen disruptor bisphenol A (BPA). Not only does BPA mess with the balance of T in your body,[37] it acts as an obesogen — a foreign chemical linked to unwanted weight gain that attaches to insulin or leptin receptors.[38] Is BPA involved in the low T that I see in my patients who are premenopausal and menopausal, in lockstep with less muscle mass, more anxiety, more depression, and a slower metabolism? We don't yet know because studies of BPA have mostly focused on its adverse effects on women who want to become pregnant and/or have polycystic ovary syndrome.

Beyond targeting individual foods that science has linked with low or high T, the Gottfried Protocol is my own secret weapon for balancing androgens, along with all the other hormones, for maximum health and vitality. In Chapter 5, I'll share a detailed plan to address key metabolic hormones — the Protocol is a combination of detoxification, ketosis, and intermittent fasting, adapted for women.

You may be thinking, "Uh, Dr. Sara, that sounds like a lot. I'm too busy." I get it, but you probably don't have time to cart around your extra 15 pounds either, or muddle through daily fatigue, or take on the downstream health problems that an unhealthy lifestyle can cause. The effort you put into this plan now will save you time — and possibly save your health — later.

## Other Ways to Boost T

Besides eating the right foods, there are other things you can do to boost T. One is to take the supplement DHEA, which as you may remember is the precursor to T, and it is sometimes used to increase T levels. For example, new research suggests that adding DHEA may maintain T levels for women on the birth control pill.[39] However, the use of DHEA is controversial because of limited information as to its long-term safety. A Cochrane database systematic review of twenty-eight randomized trials suggested that DHEA may modestly improve low sex drive, but other outcomes are lacking. Plus, so-called "androgenic" side effects are common,[40] such as oily hair and skin, acne, excessive sex drive, aggression, excessive clitoris swelling or sensitivity, excessive muscle development, male-pattern hair loss, and excess body hair. Still, given the lack of other options for raising T, I do sometimes recommend DHEA as a supplement to my patients who are unable to raise their T sufficiently with other lifestyle changes.

You might wonder if you could just start taking T in order to help the pounds melt off your middle. Or perhaps you wonder about T pellets injected under the skin. Well . . . though there are several forms of FDA-approved T treatments available to address low T in men, we lack proof that they are safe for women, which is why the FDA has not approved a T formulation for women. For now, I suggest avoiding T supplements as a treatment for women unless absolutely necessary. Hopefully, the research will catch up soon. In the meantime, commit to dietary and lifestyle changes to achieve T balance. It's safer, and still effective, without the potential side effects.

Let's go back to Nicole, from the beginning of the chapter, and her complaints of low muscle tone and sex drive, and see how she fared when she tried the Gottfried Protocol. She focused first on detoxification, then ketosis, and then added intermittent fasting. As you will see in Chapter 5, I prefer an overnight fast of fourteen to sixteen hours, but you can work your way up to it slowly. Nicole got into ketosis immediately — after her first fourteen-hour overnight fast, her blood ketones were 2.0 mmol (0.5 or greater is diagnostic of mild ketosis, which is the goal on my food plan) suggested that her metabolic flexibility would be relatively easy to restore. Within one week, her ketones were consistently at 1.0 to 2.0 mmol, suggesting that her body successfully and rapidly adapted to fat burning. After four weeks, she dropped 3 inches off her waist and 8 pounds off her weight. At that time, we found that her measures of free and total T were better, but still borderline low. I added supplemental DHEA, at a dose of 5 milligrams per day, which she purchased online. (DHEA does not require a prescription in the United States, but I recommend taking it only after consultation with an experienced clinician.). After eight weeks, she went from weighing 144 pounds down to 130, and her body fat decreased from 33 to 25 percent — giving her a normal and healthy body mass index of 23.8. She lost a total of 4 inches off her waist. Her T and DHEA went back into the normal range. Nicole felt mentally focused, her libido improved, and she was back to enjoying sex regularly. She felt healthier than she had in years — it was as if she got her body back, and her life.

## *Highlights*

▶ Testosterone (T) is a key hormone associated with weight, vitality, strength, and sex drive.

▶ Healthy men have more T than healthy women, but T is the *most abundant biologically active hormone* in women. Yes, you have more T than even estrogen.

► When women have low T, they may experience many different symptoms, such as increased weight and body fat, decreased muscle mass, declining mood, and faltering sex drive.

► Women can also have too much T, typically as part of polycystic ovary syndrome (PCOS). We need T in balance in order to function at our best.

► We know much more about low T in men than in women, but while we wait for more research, you can focus on food, lifestyle, and supplements to improve your production of T as well as other key androgens.

# 4

———

# THE KETO PARADOX

Jen is a thirty-seven-year-old woman with a stressful job in technology. She and her fiancé wanted to lose weight before their wedding, so they would look great in their photos. After hearing about the so-called miraculous ketogenic diet, they decided to try it together. Jen's main goals were to lose 15 pounds, feel trim in her wedding dress, and gain more mental clarity for planning the event. Now that you know a lot more about hormones and how they differ between men and women, can you guess what happened?

That's a trick question because first, in order to predict the outcome, you need to understand exactly what a ketogenic diet is, how it works, and why results can sometimes be paradoxical.

## KETOSIS 101

The ketogenic diet you've probably heard so much about is a low-carbohydrate, moderate-protein, high-fat diet that isn't actually new. Its first clinical application dates to more than a century ago, when it was used as a treatment for children with epilepsy. It did indeed seem like a "miracle cure" (though I would never describe anything we do in medicine as a "miracle") because in many cases, it *stopped or signifi-*

*cantly reduced* the children's seizures. About 10 to 20 percent of kids were *super responders* — they improved dramatically and early in the ketogenic process compared to other kids, and some were able to get off their seizure medication.[1] More recently, people with other neurological issues, such as multiple sclerosis, Parkinson's disease, and Alzheimer's disease, have used the ketogenic diet with success that has been reported anecdotally (there isn't yet much research on this subject).[2] Although scientists don't completely understand why this diet seems to have a beneficial effect on neurological conditions, the primary theory is that it's the ketones (also called ketone bodies).

Normally, the human body (and especially the human brain) burns sugar for energy. We get this sugar from the carbohydrates we eat (and secondarily, from the protein). When carbohydrates are drastically reduced, however, the body turns to fat for fuel instead of sugar. It does this by triggering the liver to release ketones, which the body and brain can burn and use for energy. Remember, burning fat instead of sugar is part of ketosis. We probably developed this ability early in human history, to survive the seasons when carbohydrates from fruits and vegetables were scarce or nonexistent. At such times, animal fat became a critical source of fuel, and our bodies figured out how to use it.

The brain in particular seems to thrive when fueled by ketones, not sugar. This may be why ketones (and a ketogenic diet) seem to benefit people with brain issues. Because it's easier for the body to burn sugar than ketones, burning ketones for fuel seems to induce weight loss: it takes more energy and burns more fat. Initially, weight loss was considered a side effect of ketosis (the state of burning fat instead of sugar), rather than its primary purpose.

The reason why the ketogenic diet leads to weight loss is that when you are in ketosis, you are literally burning your fat stores as fuel. When you switch to eating fewer carbs and more fat, your body recognizes that this is a new scenario. When it runs out of sugar (and glycogen, which is your liver's store of "carb energy"), your body discovers that it can rely on plenty of dietary fat coming in. This keeps your body from sensing any lack of incoming energy. There is no famine — it's just a different kind of fuel. Your body adapts, becoming metabolically flexible, and the fat on your body starts to burn away.

Getting your body to flip the switch from burning carbohydrates to burning fat offers fascinating health benefits: mental focus, better memory and attention, less inflammation, and, as I've already mentioned, weight loss. Overall, a ketogenic diet may be an easier path to weight loss because it helps you feel more satisfied than calorie-restricted diets do. Eager to lose weight, many people have been jumping on the keto bandwagon. Recently it has become a very big trend.

That all sounds great, right? But before you empty your produce bin into the trash or stock up on a year's supply of bacon, here's a reminder: *the ketogenic diet has mostly been studied in men and works quite well for them.* Women, on the other hand, tend not to do so well on this diet. There are exceptions — some women do great on keto — but in general, a man and a woman (like Jen and her fiancé) can go on an identical keto diet and get completely different results.

As we touched on earlier, keto may also not be healthy for people with different health issues. That's why if you have a history of any disease, you should speak with your physician before trying keto. If you have cancer or a history of cancer, discuss keto with your oncologist. While the majority of research on the ketogenic diet in cancer is favorable,[3] one animal model suggests that keto may worsen a certain form of cancer called acute myeloid leukemia, as published in the journal *Nature*.[4] On the other hand, most cancer cells feed on sugar, so keto may be an important tool that's synergistic to multimodal cancer prevention and treatment, though further trials are needed to explore this possibility. The bottom line: it's complicated! Keto needs to be personalized to each woman's situation. (See "Is Keto Safe for Me?" for further information on absolute and relative contraindications to the ketogenic diet.) If you have questions about keto related to particular health conditions, such as gallbladder issues or a history of kidney stones, discuss them with your healthcare professional.

## Is Keto Safe for Me?

How can you tell if the keto diet is safe for you?[5] A ketogenic diet is not safe for people who have congenital health conditions that make them unable to metabolize fatty acids. These conditions include pyruvate carboxylase deficiency, porphyria, and other fat metabolism disorders. Other health conditions that may be worsened by a ketogenic diet include pancreatitis, active gallbladder disease, impaired liver function, and poor nutritional status. It also may not be appropriate for people who have undergone gastric bypass surgery, people with a history of abdominal tumors or cancer, and those with a history of kidney failure. Those who have type 1 diabetes should avoid keto. Furthermore, I do not recommend keto for women who are pregnant or breastfeeding because of the lack of safety data.

There are also rare metabolic conditions that contraindicate the keto diet, such as carnitine deficiency (primary), carnitine palmitoyltransferase (CPT) I or II deficiency, carnitine translocase deficiency, beta-oxidation defects, mitochondrial 3-hydroxy-3-methylglutaryl-CoA synthase (mHMGS) deficiency, medium-chain acyl dehydrogenase deficiency (MCAD), long-chain acyl dehydrogenase deficiency (LCAD), short-chain acyl dehydrogenase deficiency (SCAD), long-chain 3-hydroxyacyl-CoA deficiency, and medium-chain 3-hydroxyacyl-CoA deficiency.

When in doubt, check with your doctor. It's never a bad idea to speak with your physician or health team before starting a new dietary plan. And be sure to keep up-to-date on the research as more indications and contraindications emerge, based on the latest scientific evidence.

## Keto and the Male Bias in Research

It's perhaps not surprising that women are more likely to have problems on keto, given that the bulk of the data on the ketogenic diet comes from men.[6] Some of the studies performed on men include evaluation of hunger and appetite for weight loss[7] or the time line of changes in satiety and appetite[8] in overweight and obese men;[9] studies in athletic men;[10] cardiovascular blood tests[11] in healthy men; and ketogenic tests in male (but not female) mice.[12] Similarly, low-carb diets have been mostly tested on men.[13] A small handful of ketogenic trials for weight loss have included women, but they made up less than 20 percent of the participants.[14]

This gender gap isn't unique to research on keto — or, more broadly, research on diet and nutrition. In most realms of medicine, women have historically been underrepresented in clinical research, or even left out entirely. It wasn't until the early 1990s that a federal law was passed requiring that studies funded by the National Institutes of Health (NIH) include women. Furthermore, it wasn't until 2014 that the NIH began requiring that animal studies include both sexes. *Seriously?* And it's still not routine for researchers to analyze their results by gender. Since women are not merely men with ovaries, we can't (and shouldn't) extrapolate the results of research on men to predict results in women. If we did, we would be ignoring fundamental biological differences, such as how female hormones interact with the rest of the female body, and we would be dismissing the profound endocrinological transitions that women undergo and men don't, such as pregnancy, nursing, perimenopause, and menopause.

What's more, applying something as influential as a dietary prescription to women without an adequate scientific basis can affect health and weight loss in ways that can be dangerous. Not only may women assume their failure to lose weight and feel better is their fault (and feel resentful toward their keto-successful male friends and partners), but they could end up with more risk factors for chronic disease, such as high cholesterol, inflammation, high stress, diabetes, and weight gain.

What's up? Why does keto help most men lose weight but cause some women to gain it? Furthermore, why does keto reverse some diseases, such as high blood sugar and high blood pressure, yet exacerbate others? When does keto clear inflammation, and when does keto cause it?

I've been taking care of women since 1994, but over the past ten years a large number of "keto refugees" have visited my office and participated in my online courses. I have seen up close the frustration they experience with keto—and by now, I feel like I've seen it all. Women tell me they gained weight on keto and ask if it's because of the calorie-dense food plan or the generous amount of animal fat. They experience more inflammation, their joints ache, and they wonder why they don't feel or look as great as their husbands or male co-workers using the same diet plan. They get stressed or start their period and come out of ketosis.

We aren't totally sure why women respond to keto differently than men do,[15] but I can make an educated guess, based on what I've seen in my practice (and you've read about in the past three chapters): *it's the hormones.* From a hormonal perspective, it's logical that a diet low in carbs and high in fat would have a different effect on men than on women. As you learned in the previous chapter, the endocrine system, and the hormones it produces, responds differently to fat, carbs, and protein, and since women and men have very different hormonal profiles, of course their bodies and hormones will react to a ketogenic diet differently.

So let's go back to Jen and her fiancé. What do you think happened when they both changed to a food plan low in carbs, moderate in protein, and high in fat?

# HORMONES, FAT STORAGE, AND THE (DIET) BATTLE OF THE SEXES

As you may have guessed by this point, Jen's fiancé quickly lost weight: 12 pounds in the first ten days on keto. Jen, on the other hand, *gained weight* almost immediately and noticed no change at all in her brain fog. This was not what she expected. Frustrated and disillusioned, she gave up on keto. But when you keep hearing how great something is, it's hard not to give it another try. Jen began to wonder if she had "done keto right." After all, she admittedly hadn't been tracking her carb, protein, and fat grams (her macronutrients, or "macros"), so maybe she wasn't hitting the right ratios.

Six months later, Jen tried keto again. This time, she faithfully kept a log of her food in order to stick to the proper macronutrient rations that she'd read about online: 10 percent carb, 20 percent protein, and 70 percent fat. But now she had a new problem: she was always hungry. Keto is meant to kill your appetite, so Jen couldn't understand why that wasn't happening. Her fiancé wasn't hungry. He'd have some bacon and eggs and feel great (and then be down another pound!). But that feeling of satisfaction never kicked in for Jen, and things got even worse during her period, when she craved chocolate cake. After one month, she didn't feel any different (other than constantly dreaming about bread and doughnuts), and while she hadn't gained any weight, she hadn't lost any either. Frustrated again, she quit. When she finally came to see me, Jen told me all about her disappointing experience, and I reassured her that she was definitely not the only woman to struggle with keto. Then I told her not to give up hope just yet.

Why is this happening to so many women? What is it about female hormones that respond so differently to keto? First of all, it's helpful to look at the science of dieting in general. Women are already, sorry to say, at a disadvantage when it comes to weight loss. Studies have demonstrated that on a diet, men lose more weight than women do.[16] One study showed that they lost twice as much weight and three times as much fat mass when compared to women on a diet.[17] Men seem to lose more belly fat (the more dangerous visceral fat), while women tend to lose more subcutaneous fat (the less harmful type).[18] That translates to more metabolic improvement in men (the rate at which their bodies transform food into fuel).

The differences go even further. Men tend to be less likely to be aware of their weight or dissatisfied with their weight, and they are less likely to even try to lose weight — and of course, when they did try, according to one study, they were 40 percent more likely than women to lose and maintain a weight loss greater than 10 pounds and increase their exercise over the course of one year.[19]

By contrast, women are more likely to want a lower body weight than men do and consistently have higher levels of body dissatisfaction.[20] Unrealistic societal norms and the multi-billion-dollar dieting industry affect women more than men. There is even a ripple effect related to income. Waist circumference is negatively correlated with wages for women but not for men. *No obesity measure correlates with men's earnings.*[21] Clearly, women experience a greater burden when it comes to weight loss.

## Weighty Issues

Another issue that women face more commonly than men do is food addiction and other eating disorders. Overeating is the most common one. Women have a fourfold greater risk of being addicted to food — we are more likely to eat for emotional reasons, positive or negative, or because we feel overly stressed. That means that for us, giving up the cupcakes may not be a straightforward undertaking. This factor makes compliance with any diet, let alone a low-carb diet, more challenging. As a woman, I know these pressures well, and I have internalized many of them. Together we will keep an eye on health, not just appearance, because that's my primary job as a precision medicine physician.

It all seems terribly unfair, I know. And it is! But it is also one of the main reasons why I developed the Gottfried Protocol and wrote this book. I want to help level the playing field with an accessible, user-friendly approach that can help women succeed on keto as well as men do. The Gottfried Protocol works *with* your hormones, instead of forcing on your body a program that wasn't tested on women or designed with your body chemistry in mind. When you are able to get healthy on your own terms, you'll gain the confidence, clarity, energy, and good health that will enable you to thrive.

## THE SCIENCE OF FEMALE HORMONES AND KETO

Before I explain why your hormones will work well with the Gott-fried Protocol, let's take a deeper dive into why female hormones don't work with traditional keto diets. Let's start with Jen. Jen's ketogenic diet "failures" and the ensuing frustrations were likely due to her hormones and unresolved inflammation. To confirm this, the first thing I did was order some tests. We discovered that Jen had several issues:

1. Jen had a high level of cortisol in her urine, which mirrored her concern that she was under a lot of stress. Many women of Jen's age experience high perceived stress and become so accustomed to the feeling that they don't even realize it's a problem. But chronic stress can be a primary cause of brain fog, concentration issues, high blood pressure, and subclinical hypothalamic-pituitary-adrenal dysfunction (so-called adrenal fatigue, a term I don't like). Remember that Jen was eating low-carb. Since high-quality whole-food carbohydrates like greens and multicolored vegetables can promote healthy adrenal function and stabilize cortisol levels, I suspected her diet could be exacerbating her stress.

2. She had high blood sugar, in the range that indicated prediabetes, a condition in which blood sugar is above

normal but not quite at diabetes level. Prediabetes is generally considered to be a warning that diabetes is imminent without treatment; it is a telltale sign of metabolic inflexibility. (See Notes for laboratory criteria.[22]) Prediabetes is common in overweight women and even in some women who are not overweight but can no longer process carbohydrates efficiently or who have become insulin resistant. High blood sugar can also cause concentration issues and a general feeling of being unwell. It's also a risk factor for heart disease, although some women have no symptoms (but all the risks). Jen was surprised that she could have high blood sugar while eating low-carb, but for some women, certain types of fat can actually trigger high blood sugar.[23] I've seen this in Jen as well as other patients. Low carb doesn't always mean lower blood sugar — saturated fat may raise blood sugar levels, perhaps due to inflammation.

3. Jen's thyroid, T, and growth hormone were borderline low. I suspected this was also a function of her low-carb diet, since carbohydrates can also promote healthier thyroid and estrogen function in many women.

4. Another test showed that Jen had chronic inflammation. We hear a lot about inflammation, usually in the context of its being a bad thing that can contribute to weight gain. Typically, that means the immune system is having a dysfunctional response to a perceived injury or infection. But because there's a lot that's misunderstood about inflammation, it's helpful to unpack the concept. There are two types: a short-term type of inflammation, called acute, and a long-term type of inflammation, called chronic. Acute inflammation occurs when you cut yourself or sprain an ankle or get an infection, and in such a case the acute inflammation (immune response) is good — the region becomes swollen and red as your white blood cells swarm in and fight for your healing. Jen, however, showed evidence of chronic inflammation (an immune response that won't resolve), as indicated by a high level of c-reactive protein

in her blood. Sometimes this is caused by too much saturated fat in women,[24] though the science is still evolving and suggests that lifestyle factors, such as exercise, may play a role.[25]

This list gives you a sense of the specific ways in which a typical ketogenic diet won't work very well for women with hormonal imbalance. Traditional keto may be too low in carbohydrates for women with a hormone imbalance, since carbs help mitigate the stress response and lower cortisol. They also boost growth hormone and support thyroid function.

Another issue is inflammation, specifically chronic inflammation. Chronic or unresolved inflammation is problematic and can have a variety of causes. Sometimes it's due to an immune response that never turns off, like a light left on in a room. That can occur when you eat inflammatory foods (refined carbohydrates, sugary drinks, certain fried foods), or because of exposure to toxins, chronic stress, excess visceral fat, and even autoimmune diseases like Hashimoto's thyroiditis. Chronic and unresolved inflammation is nothing to mess around with as it can lead to other consequences, such as heart disease, Alzheimer's disease, cancer, and depression.

One study showed that the shift into ketosis, by which fat is burned preferentially during exercise, takes longer to kick in for women as compared to men. Men tend to burn fat more easily, and they burn it at a lower intensity than women. I believe this is because women's bodies not only tend to need more carbs and hang on to fat for a variety of reasons (including fertility, though the problem persists and may worsen after menopause), but because women tend to have a more inflammatory response to certain fats. Because of this, their bodies resist the switch to fat burning longer than men's bodies do. That inflammatory response from fats can also elevate blood sugar, as it seemed to have done with Jen.

## What's Your Metabolotype?
## Apple, Pear, or Celery?

*Where* a woman stores her fat seems to be a good predictor
of how her physiology behaves — storing fat predominantly
in the abdominal area carries with it the same metabolic
risks that it does for men, especially those who have obesity.
However, many women with obesity and "pear-shaped" fat
stores are actually *protected* from metabolic and cardiovascular
diseases.

We can call these different metabolic types *metabolotypes*.
Beyond the apple (extra fat at the waist) and the pear (extra fat
at the hips and thighs — that's me!), there's the celery (no extra
fat). These are the lucky women who just don't gain weight.
They have a fast metabolism no matter what. Lifelong athletes
often fit into this category — my youngest sister is one of them.
She just never struggles with her weight, even after reaching
age forty and having two kids.

On the other hand, women are also much more efficient
at storing fat compared to men. After eating a high-calorie,
high-fat meal, women with pear-shaped fat distributions store
more of the fat in the gluteo-femoral region — the good old
butt and thighs. As I mentioned in the Metabolic Hormone
Questionnaire in Chapter 1, you can determine if you have an
apple or pear shape by measuring your waist-to-hip ratio. If
your waist measurement divided by your hip measurement is
greater than 0.85 for women, or greater than 0.90 for men, you
have an apple shape.

Whether you have an apple or pear metabolotype, there
is a way to customize the Gottfried Protocol for you. In my
experience, apples need more detoxification, fewer carbs (at
least temporarily, for four weeks), deeper ketosis (where you
are producing significant levels of ketones from burning fat,
defined as greater than 1.0 mmol/L), and intermittent fasting.
(Remember Melissa from Chapter 1? She has reduced her waist-
to-hip measurement from 0.92 to 0.88, and is on her way to

> better health and lower risk of metabolic syndrome, diabetes, and heart disease. Small changes can truly aggregate to major transformation.) Pears can get away with lighter ketosis (where you are producing a mild amount of ketones from burning fat, defined as a level of 0.5–1.0 mmol/L) but also respond well to intermittent fasting. In Part 2, we will perform measurements to check your metabolotype, and I'll provide additional prescriptions to personalize the Gottfried Protocol.

So, what's the verdict? Is keto out for Jen (and for you)? Definitely not. While classic keto may not work for most women, I've found that with certain work-arounds specifically designed for a woman's body and hormonal profile, keto *can absolutely* work for women. What's more, women with either the apple or the pear shape can succeed with a well-formulated ketogenic diet—the trick is the "well-formulated" part.

## THE GOTTFRIED PROTOCOL: A PROGRAM FOR METABOLIC FLEXIBILITY

Watching how these symptoms, test results, and reactions to keto have played out in my practice has formed the foundation for my plan. Over the past decade, I've tackled the keto paradox with a smart, safe protocol that, based on my research, has been proved to work for women. Now I'm sharing it with you.[26] I'm going to give you an evidence-based way to enter mild ketosis that activates your get-me-lean hormones, reverses inflammation, and provides you with peace of mind regarding safety and effectiveness. You'll learn the tips and tricks that I've discovered while taking care of women on keto, such as when you might need a few blood tests and how to prep meals so keto works in your busy life. Here are other key features of this female-centric plan:

1. Detoxifying before and during keto, which can balance hormones by freeing up your endocrine system from the onslaught of a toxic load.
2. Understanding which dietary adjustments to make based on your body type.
3. Layering in specific carbohydrates that feed the beneficial microbes in the gut (your microbiome) and also the endocrine system in a way that further balances hormones.
4. Incorporating intermittent fasting into your regimen, which can keep you in mild ketosis with a slightly higher carbohydrate intake.
5. Timing your largest and smallest meals the right way, so you never end up starving and overeating.

In Part 2, I'll guide you through the complete four-week protocol, with recommendations for personalizing the ketogenic diet for your situation, body type, and lifestyle — just as I do with my precision medicine patients. We will cover the do's and don'ts of the protocol, and I'll provide a troubleshooting guide, shopping list, and recipes that I developed in my own kitchen. Along the way, I'll share scientific breakthroughs that will help you succeed, such as how to make up your sleep debt, which has been shown to simultaneously help multiple hormones, including insulin, cortisol, ghrelin, and leptin.[27]

And what about Jen? She followed the very same plan I outline in this book. She started on the Gottfried Protocol, eating more organic vegetables than she did in the first two (unsuccessful) rounds of keto, along with supplements that addressed an overburdened liver — that is, a liver that doesn't detoxify chemicals efficiently, which may contribute to inflammation and foil attempts at weight loss.

Next, Jen added intermittent fasting to the plan. She ate between 8 a.m. and 6 p.m. and went to bed earlier. After two weeks of adjusting to intermittent fasting without hijacking her cortisol, she progressed to a 16:8 protocol, which means that she ate between 10 a.m. and 6 p.m. She stopped eating three hours before she went to sleep. After an overnight fast, she was ready for a healthy breakfast with some whole-food carbs, such as avocado on keto toast.

Jen prepped meals on the weekend, so that her refrigerator and freezer were stocked with nourishing soups and snacks that fed her gut microbes, lowered her insulin, and were rich in plant-based fats — yet made it easy to stick to the plan during the busy workweek. (See the recipes in Chapter 9.) She restricted animal-based fats to less than 30 percent of her daily total fat intake but continued to enjoy wild meats, such as a bison burger wrapped in lettuce or grass-fed beef such as filet mignon on the grill, and she cooked with ghee, olive oil, and avocado oil.

She learned about medium-chain triglycerides (MCTs) — a special type of fat you'll read about in Chapter 5 — that helps produce ketones, boost fat burning, and ignite brain function. (The "medium-chain" refers to how the carbon atoms are arranged in their chemical structure — most fats in a typical diet are long-chain triglycerides.) MCT oil can help you stay in ketosis (fat-burning mode), even if you add a few more carbs to your diet. Jen added MCTs to her salads and smoothies, along with macadamia nuts as a snack, and she ate more fatty fish at dinner.

In four weeks, she lost 12 pounds, most of it fat, and she felt better than she had in years. Her prediabetes and brain fog disappeared. *Success!* She was delighted. And she's kept the weight off. For long-term maintenance, she cycles in and out of the Gottfried Protocol, a mashup of a low-carb Mediterranean diet and detoxification, ketosis, and intermittent fasting.

Before Jen started the Gottfried Protocol, we got clear about her values. I asked her to write a personal value statement regarding her goals, hormones, and weight. Here is Jen's statement:

Scary diseases run in my family, like diabetes and heart disease. I believe that I will not develop these diseases if I choose a lifestyle that won't allow them to take hold. That means being careful with what I eat and how much alcohol I drink. I want to be fit and lean so that I fit into my wedding dress, but beyond that, I want to show up for my marriage as the healthiest version of myself. My relationship is my highest value — my relationship to my husband and myself. My career is next, and I have to be the best version of myself to be successful and create financial independence. All of these values stem from my health.

Jen used her personal values statement as a simple framework to guide her behavior during the four weeks of the Gottfried Protocol. She wrote her statement on a sticky note, placed it on her bathroom mirror, and reread it while brushing her teeth and flossing. It became a lighthouse for her, a beacon in the sunshine and storm of life.

You, like Jen, *can* be successful on a ketogenic diet. In Part 2, you'll learn exactly how. This protocol is designed for a new generation of women seeking health, a good life with the occasional carb, and a closet full of clothes that fit. In the following pages, I'll give you all the tools you need to burn stubborn fat, gain energy, clear that brain fog, and lower your chances of developing a chronic disease. All this awaits you, and the answer, after all, really can be keto. But it's not going to be a man's keto. It's going to be all yours.

## *Highlights*

Ketogenic diets have many proven benefits, including mental focus, reduced appetite, and weight loss, although most studies of the diet have focused on men.

▶ We must deal with the keto paradox: the diet that works well for men often doesn't work well for women.

▶ Though we do not completely understand the sex and gender differences in diet effectiveness, fat distribution, and fat type between men and women, the answers seem to be rooted in the differences in hormones.

▶ The reasons women don't generally seem to benefit from the traditional ketogenic diet have to do with hormones, which can influence detoxification, stress and cortisol, thyroid function, hunger and food addiction, and low blood sugar.

▶ Eating crappy carbs can spike your insulin and blood sugar, leading to insulin block and fat accumulation. Alternatively, eating more healthy fat makes you feel satisfied, and it slows down or eliminates the rise in blood sugar rise that many foods cause.

▶ This book describes a modified ketogenic diet and lifestyle plan specifically formulated for women and personalized to your particular body type. You can succeed at keto!

# PART II

# The Four-Week Gottfried Protocol

# 5

## HOW TO START AND WHAT TO EAT

Are you ready to change the way you look and feel, not just by improving the fit of your skinny jeans today but by improving the expression of your genes for the rest of your life? It all starts with your food and how it communicates with your hormones — changing your diet gives you the true power to reset your hormones and amplify fat loss. It's the change you've been waiting for: major improvements in health and wellness that I witness daily in my patients. I'm sharing them with you now. You've learned about the important hormones in the symphony, and now you're ready to orchestrate greater metabolic flexibility.

Though changing food habits can be remarkably difficult, it's well worth it: the hormonal changes you'll enjoy will be dramatic. I have evidence-based tactics to help you overcome the challenge of changing what you eat; I'll share these proven techniques in this chapter and beyond. This chapter covers the nuts and bolts you'll need to prepare for the first week of the protocol — and the first week of your new, healthier life.

## HOW CHANGE STARTS

For the Gottfried Protocol, limiting carbohydrates over the short term will instigate a change in the body's hormonal messaging. After four weeks, we'll increase slow-burn carbohydrates over the long term to prevent difficulties that some people experience on extreme keto diets.

This time line is based on sound scientific reasoning. First, we want your hormones to scream loud and clear that it's time to raid the reserves, empty the pantry, and prepare the body for a state of equilibrium rather than fat storage. Cutting out carbohydrates is the best way to inspire this message, but we want to do it in a way that is easy on your body and optimizes hormonal balance. To do this, the Gottfried Protocol starts with a detox, then activates the powerful weight-loss power of traditional ketogenic diets, and finally harnesses the health-boosting and disease-resistant qualities of the Mediterranean diet for the long term. The Protocol features a three-stage, four-week program with a built-in self-assessment so you can adjust the program depending on how your unique body responds. Here's a rundown of the features that make the Gottfried Protocol different from other plans:

- Detoxification early in the process to support the body as it rids itself of stored toxins as fat is melted off.
- Scaled carbohydrate recommendations, beginning with the most restrictive, to encourage hormones to signal fat burning and a metabolism that supports long-term weight loss.
- Increasing slow-burn carbohydrate consumption in the second and third phases (Transition and Integration) to avoid the potential long-term issues associated with extremely low-carb diets.

This plan has been carefully constructed to work with a woman's body in a healthy and effective way. This approach includes these key benefits:

- Significant reduction of abdominal fat, which reduces inflammation and helps sustain growth hormone balance. Remember, in Chapter 1 we talked about how increased abdominal fat plays a greater role than age does in the decline of growth hormone. Perhaps even more important, for our goals, growth hormone levels are *improved* with weight loss.[1]
- Monitoring your unique body to see how you respond to a low-carbohydrate diet. Not everyone will respond in the same way, and you'll want to be able to adjust the Gottfried Protocol to make sure it is right for you.

## FOOD HABITS
## CAN BE CHANGED

Okay, I get it—all of this sounds great in theory. But I know what you're wondering: let's get down to the details. What exactly does this change of diet look like . . . and how hard will it be?

For many people, food is more than just fuel: it has a powerful emotional and psychological hold over us. Does the crunch of chips dipped in guacamole remind you of a perfect summer day? (Are you thinking "Where's my margarita?") Does a gooey-fluffy chocolate croissant arouse memories of a trip to France? Maybe it's simply a hearty bowl of pasta that takes you back to happy times around the family table growing up? Whatever your personal favorites, I get it: the power of food is rooted in memory, good times, and the strong desire to re-create the sensation associated with these positive experiences.

Memories can be both dangerous and instructive when you head into a new diet. Over the past five years, scientific research has been shedding light on how memory plays a powerful role in a range of risky behaviors, including use of hard-core drugs, binge eating, compulsive use of video games, excessive consumption of alcohol, use (and misuse) of marijuana, compulsive shopping, and constant internet surfing. The culprit, as revealed in this research, is not always the activity or substance, but rather the type of decision making involved. What was once a conscious decision to engage in an activity has been transformed into a subconscious one by means of what researchers call *habit memories*.[2] A multidisciplinary team of scientists from universities around the globe theorizes that rogue habit learning is one of the keys to explaining the entire process of addictive behaviors.[3]

Think of habit memories as a mental bias that makes changing food behaviors especially tough.[4] Fortunately, according to the latest research, we can learn how to overcome this type of mental interference and improve our decision making. We can extinguish habit memories.[5]

I believe women are particularly vulnerable to habit memories, and they can create unique challenges related to our hormones, metabolism, and weight loss. The research confirms my hunch.[6] Full disclosure: I used to be one of those women. My habit memory was eating chocolate chip cookies with my grandmother as a kid. Cookies were a source of comfort for me, and my go-to treat when stressed, until I learned better ways of soothing myself, like texting or calling a friend, doing yoga, practicing meditation, and exercising. I learned how to rewrite habit memories in order to honor my female biology, and so can you.

This means that when you're looking at a simple choice — like whether to have a cup of herbal tea or a pint of ice cream after dinner — your deepest desires and decision making may be based on habit memories. And we know what your habit memory would choose! However, your hormones see the situation differently. Every food you eat becomes a real-time driver of function, such as good health and high energy levels — or dysfunction, such as a thickening waistline or a depressing number on the bathroom scale. Fortunately, your taste buds turn over every two weeks, so as you enter ketosis and start losing weight, you will form new memories of healthy foods that support your lean hormones.

# BUT FIRST . . . WHY?

One of the best ways to change your food habits is to get clear on your personal values and write a statement expressing them. This statement can become a touchstone that you return to over the next four weeks and beyond. It doesn't have to be complicated: simply write a few bulleted points or sentences about *why* you want to lose weight and how this desire relates to your beliefs and values. Be specific about the people and situations that make you feel most alive. Here are a few prompts:

- My goals for weight loss are . . .
- The reason I want to lose weight is . . .
- This is important to me because . . .
- So that I can . . .

In Chapter 4, I shared Jen's personal value statement. When I asked Lara to create one, she shared a poignant story:

> The day before I started the Gottfried Protocol, I was with my children and we were taking slow-motion videos of us each blowing dandelion seeds. When I saw the videos of me in profile view, I just wanted to cry. I deleted the videos. My mom never wanted to be in a picture because she was ashamed of her appearance, even though she was thin and beautiful. I don't want to miss out on those family moments and memories, and I want to feel confident about showing up in those family photos. And I want to make sure I'm modeling healthy attitudes about body image to my kids.

From this story, Lara wrote the following personal value statement:

> To be the best version of myself, to honor my power to determine my health destiny by combatting my genetic risk for diabetes and Alzheimer's disease through a healthy lifestyle, to appreciate life

and people for the gifts that they are, and to help others fully realize their potential in life and health.

Before you embark on this plan, take some time to write your own personal value statement. Think about what you're hoping to achieve —and, most important, *why* these goals matter to you. This values statement will keep you motivated as you embrace this new way of eating and living: and it will be a reminder you can turn to again and again over the coming weeks, whenever you need motivation.

## From Dr. Sara's Case Files

Caroline is a forty-four-year-old woman who lost 50 pounds following the Gottfried Protocol. Once I showed her the basics, she was off and running. When I first met her, she was 5 feet, 8 inches tall, and weighed 200 pounds. She lost 35 pounds in her first six months of cycling through the Gottfried Protocol, and 15 more pounds over the next six months. Her main tips for success are to have a freezer full of soups and stews, to make lunch the main meal of the day (and not just a tiny salad, but a satisfying meal with plenty of plant-based fat), and to avoid snacks. Most important were meal prep and storing food in the correct portion sizes. When she fit back into her high school jeans, she explained that her hormones were back on track too: her heavy periods (a sign of estrogen dominance) had resolved, and her night sweats (a sign of insulin block and possibly fluctuating estrogen) had disappeared. She had renewed energy for exercising outside, including jogging with her dog.

## HOW FOOD AND HORMONES COMMUNICATE

As we get started on the course for better hormonal and metabolic function, let's connect the dots between your food and your hormones. Once you understand how food directly impacts your hormones (and hence your weight), we will dive into the how-to, and I'll share the four-week hormone reset that has helped hundreds of women take charge of their health. In this next section, you'll get actionable advice and specific dietary guidelines so that you can put your newfound knowledge into practice.

Savory tortilla chips, a freshly baked pastry, and comforting pasta are wildly different foods, right? Not if you ask your hormones or your metabolism. All of those foods, once eaten, turn into pretty much the same thing: processed carbohydrates mixed with fat that hold almost zero nutritional value yet trigger a boatload of inflammation. If I eat one serving of these foods (and it's hard for me to stop at just one), I can guarantee that my weight will be up the next day. For your hormones, these favorite foods transform into something far more sinister — a message that tells your body to store fat.

I know it's not easy to give up some of your favorites — after all, these foods are connected to habit memories. We have emotional and psychological connections with our childhood favorites and our go-to comfort foods. Not to mention that they taste good! Say you are going down the buffet line. Where you expect to see the label "Fettuccine Alfredo," you see one that says "Store-More-Fat-Hormone Pasta." Would you take a serving?

To your hormones, food isn't flavor, texture, and happy memories; to your hormones, food is information. The complex conversation between food and hormones is the main reason why the ketogenic diet works differently for women versus men. In Part 1, you read about how hormones work and how different aspects of food influence them — now is the time to eat in a way that honors and respects these crucial food-hormone connections.

Here's the beautiful part: because food is information, we can use food choices to communicate with our hormones in the way we desire. Once you learn the language of hormones, you'll be able to guide the conversation. If you're carrying extra weight or body fat, it's almost certainly because those hormones have been receiving very little in the way of encouragement. So now we're going to use food to tell them, loud and clear, that this is their time to thrive.

To do this, the Gottfried Protocol progresses through stages, each one allowing more satisfying and less restrictive food selections.

## OVERVIEW OF THE FOUR-WEEK GOTTFRIED PROTOCOL

After years of leading women through a ketogenic diet designed to honor their hormones, I realized that most of us need to think of keto as a short-term pulse, not a long-term diet involving lifelong restricted eating. Trial and error have shown that four weeks may be the ideal length for a ketogenic pulse for women. After you complete your first four-week pulse, I'll show you how to rotate in and out of keto, using intermittent fasting and carb cycling so that you can gain all of the hormone benefits of keto without the problems that so many women face. The key point is to commit to four weeks (Prep plus Implementation) of eating in a way that serves you, followed by another phase (Transition) in which we test your carb limit and see your response to immune-triggering foods. Here is the basic time line:

**Preparation**
20–25 grams of net carbs and detoxification. Keep a ketogenic ratio of 2:1. Get your bowels moving so you can mobilize fat!

**Implementation**
20–25 grams net carbs per day, and add intermittent fasting (14/10 to 16/8). Continue a ketogenic ratio of 2:1.

**Transition**
Start to add net carbs slowly, 5 grams at a time, and heading toward a ketogenic ratio of 1:1 for the long term, or until you repeat the diet.

- **Preparation (seven days).** This week sets the foundation for your body to release toxins as the Gottfried Protocol starts melting fat. Toxins are pollutants, synthetic chemicals, heavy metals, and endocrine disruptors that are stored in fat tissue, mess with your hormones, and make you store excess fat. (This release of toxins is one of the reasons why many people feel lousy on traditional ketogenic diets.) To put it less delicately, you must be pooping every day to clear out the toxins and process the healthy fat you'll be burning. You'll take a detox questionnaire to guide you as you improve your detoxification pathways. You'll be eating more of the vegetables known for their toxin-binding capacity, such as bok choy, broccoli, broccoli sprouts, cauliflower, and kale. Along the way, we will wrangle with those fat-storing hormones (such as cortisol, insulin, and leptin), which have been running the show, by introducing intermittent fasting, which is covered in the next chapter. Third, we will jump-start growth hormone, testosterone, and other metabolic hormones by feeding you the dietary sources needed to produce more of them.

- **Implementation (twenty-one days).** This three-week period is designed to trigger weight loss while boosting energy, gut health, and metabolic hormones, so it will include the right amount of slow-burning carbohydrates. The focus will be on dialing in the right amount of variety, nutrient density, and quantity of food for you.

At the end of twenty-eight days, you'll complete a self-assessment to help you adjust the protocol by finding your body's optimal macronutrient balance, which will encourage healthy weight loss.

- **Transition (variable).** Once you've completed the core four-week program, you'll begin the process called Transition. This is when you will slowly add back some key good carbs, in increments of 5 grams every three days. This stage includes additional detoxification support to help your body rid itself of the toxins released from fat over the previous weeks. Most important, Transition is a time of celebrating your new body, the improved communication between your diet and hormones, and even a new set of healthier habit memories. Where's my cheesy zoodle ragu? Yum!

Look, I know this may seem like a lot of detail to keep track of, or it may sound complicated. But don't stress; we will go through this one step at a time. And you'll find that these baby steps add up to major transformation. You might be thinking—can't I just take a drug? Or start peptides to boost my growth hormone? Or take up kickboxing? I wish it were that simple, but the truth is that food is the primary driver of your weight and health. Dial in the food, and we can dial in the weight that is the healthiest for you.

## Getting Started in Three Steps

1. Know How Your Hormones React to Your Food
2. Be the Guinea Pig
3. Count Your Macros

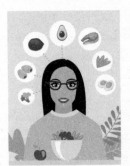 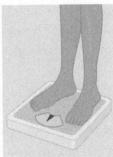 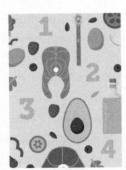

**Know** How Your Hormones React to Your Food

**Be** the Guinea Pig

**Count** Your Macros

## THE BASICS, STEP BY STEP

Before we get into the specific foods for each stage, let's consider the basics, one step at a time.

## Step 1: Know How Your
## Hormones React to Your Food

The first step is to consider how your hormones interpret food as information. The best example is sugar (that is, refined carbohydrate —see the box "Understand Your Macronutrients"), which sends one of two messages. If your hormones determine that your body needs the sugar at that moment, your hormonal system will communicate to your metabolism that the sugar should be packaged up as blood glucose and released into the bloodstream to be burned. However, if your hormones determine that your body doesn't need the sugar (and, by the way, it *never* needs the 152 pounds of table sugar, plus additional refined carbohydrates, that Americans tend to eat each year), your hormonal system will signal to the body's energy-processing system (metabolism) that the sugar (or carbs) should be converted to fat and stored.

Based on this concept, it might seem that if we ate only the amount of sugar and carbs that we need to burn each day, we wouldn't gain weight, right? Energy in, energy out. In a perfectly working body, that would be true, but who has one of those? Many of us have spent a lifetime abusing our hormones with fast-burning carbohydrates, so our systems get stuck in store-the-sugar mode.

The interplay between metabolism, hormones, and food intake is incredibly complex and not well understood, but we do know that certain foods trigger hormonal messages that cause the body to pack on weight—exactly what you don't want. Other foods trigger hormonal messages that tell the body to burn the fat reserves—exactly what you do want. We also know that not everyone responds the same way to food messages; as you learned in Chapter 3, sex and even gender differences can be profound. Not only that, but individual differences owing to genetics, food sensitivities, and toxic load can be even greater. (Regarding genetic response to food, the gene-environment interface can modulate ketones, cholesterol, cognitive function, weight loss, and how you adapt to fat burning, which we will cover later.) The way that food and your body interact is just like conversation: context and audience are everything. Comment to your best friend about your bad boss while exercising at the gym, and you both get a good laugh; say the same thing to your co-workers during a team meeting and you might find yourself looking for a new job.

## Understand Your Macronutrients

The Gottfried Protocol is a four-week program with a specific macronutrient pattern: low carbohydrate, moderate protein, and high fat. Carbs, protein, and fat are all different forms of fuel for the body — here's a quick refresher on their functions, along with an overview of targets to hit for success on this plan.

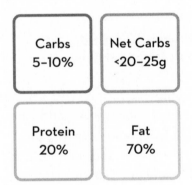

| Carbs | Net Carbs |
|-------|-----------|
| 5–10% | <20–25g |
| Protein | Fat |
| 20% | 70% |

### Carbs
- Carbs turn into sugar in your body.
- These nutrients provide 4 calories of energy per 1 gram.
- Your need for carbs depends on your exercise level. For example, women at the higher end of the range, those avid, high-intensity exercisers who work out six hours per week or more, should eat about 35–50 grams of carbs each day.
- Carbs are important! Don't malign them: we need carbs for optimal thyroid and adrenal function. But too much isn't a good thing either. We need to determine your carb limit for

weight loss and hormone balance: high enough to support the thyroid and adrenal glands but low enough to repair your levels of insulin, leptin, growth hormone, and testosterone.

### Net Carbs
- Net carbs are simply the carbohydrates absorbed by the body.
- Calculate net carbs for whole foods by taking the total carb count and subtracting the grams of fiber.[7]
- Aim for 25 grams of net carbs each day. This is essential, especially for women, to feed the microbiome and to stay in balance while on a ketogenic diet. (Read more on page 121.)

## Protein
- Protein helps build and repair muscle, but it can turn into sugar (via a process called gluconeogenesis) if you eat too much of it.
- It provides 4 calories of energy per 1 gram.
- Aim for 50–75 grams of protein per day. Some of my patients need to remain at the lower end of the limit (50–60 grams) to avoid problems with blood sugar and stay in ketosis.

## Fat
- Fat helps you make healthy hormones.
- It provides 9 calories of energy per 1 gram.
- Aim for 60 to 90 grams of healthy fat per day.

## Step 2: Be the Guinea Pig

This plan provides a solid framework to follow, but it's also designed for personalization. The key to using the messaging power of food to your advantage is to pay attention to your unique body's response as you use the program. The goal is to learn how to speak to *your* hormones, practicing the principles of precision medicine, in order to lose weight and overcome unhealthy habit memories.

First, we have to reprogram your hormonal messaging system to tell your body to burn fat reserves rather than add to them. This is where personalized nutrition becomes really important—for example, you will define the daily carbohydrate level that works best to support your health. If you have insulin block or carb intolerance, getting the sugar and carbs down will be key to your success. You may not know if these are issues are relevant to you unless you've been previously diagnosed with prediabetes or if you struggle with weight loss (by detecting excess deep belly fat through body composition testing, the lab testing described in the Notes, or stalling in your weight-loss efforts on the Gottfried Protocol.)[8] Many people with insulin block have to temporarily limit even healthy carbs, such as certain fruits and starchy vegetables. We will personalize your intake of protein and fat too, but carbs come first.

Second, we want to measure your results accurately, so you can be accountable to yourself and continue on the path to success. It's all too easy to fall back on subjective measures of progress. For example, here's how my mind works sometimes: If I wear pants that make me feel fat, if I am grumpy after a poor night's sleep, or if I catch a view of myself in the mirror that I don't like, I might be tricked into believing that I have failed at weight loss and come down with a case of the "f*ck its." (More on this in the next chapter.) On the other hand, a flattering comment or a long hike might make me think I deserve to cheat on my program. But if I measure progress through clear metrics, my assessment won't be based on my mood or my clothing choices but on a series of inarguably objective data points. (That's where measuring your progress and personalizing your program come in.)

Before starting the program, measure your waist circumference, hip circumference, and weight. You can then calculate your body mass index (BMI) based on your weight and height—the healthy goal is a BMI of 18.5 to 24.9 $m/kg^2$. For women who aren't satisfied with this range, I get it: studies show that the ideal BMI of 22–24.9 is associated with the lowest risk of premature mortality.[9] You can also divide waist circumference by hip circumference to get your waist-to-hip ratio. Follow these steps:

- Measure your waist at the height of your belly button.
- Measure your hips by finding the largest circumference while holding the measuring tape level.
- Measure your weight first thing in the morning, on an empty stomach, ideally after you've pooped (that is, completely evacuated your bowels).
- Record these measurements in the "Measuring Success" table. This table includes room for additional stats that you may want to track, such as your net carbs or fasting blood sugar.
  - Your waist-to-hip ratio is your waist circumference (in inches or centimeters) divided by your hip circumference (measured in the same units).
  - You can determine your BMI with a calculator you can find online or with this formula: BMI = weight ÷ height$^2$. If you use kilograms and centimeters, you have your result. If you use pounds and inches, you need to multiply the result by 703. (See Notes for more details, including an online calculator.)[10] For example, for a woman who weighs 155 pounds with a height of 5 feet 4 inches (64 inches total), BMI = $(155 \div 64^2) \times 703 = 26.6$ m/kg$^2$.
  - Your metabolotype may vary over time. If your waist-to-hip ratio is greater than 0.85 (the measure is 0.9 for men), you have an apple metabolotype. If your waist measures 2 inches or more than your hips measure, you are definitely an apple. If your hips are larger than your waist and your BMI is 25 or greater, there's a good chance you have a pear metabolotype. If your BMI is less than 20 and your waist measures less than your hips, there's a good chance you have a celery metabolotype. (Bust size, whether large or small, doesn't really matter in terms of metabolism. We are primarily interested in your waist-to-hip measurement.) Write your metabolotype in the space provided in the table—it may change over the four weeks of the program!

## Measuring Success: Before and After Measurements

|  | Before | After |
|---|---|---|
| Waist (inches or centimeters) | | |
| Hips (inches or centimeters | | |
| Weight (pounds or kilograms) | | |
| Waist-to-hip ratio (WHR) | | |
| Body mass index (BMI) | | |
| Metabolotype | | |
| Other | | |

For more advanced measurements, see the Notes.[11]

Finally, "being the guinea pig" means testing whether you're making ketones. As you'll learn in the next chapter, it's the best way to measure your success with getting into ketosis.

## Step 3: Count Your Macros

This part gets confusing for a lot of people, so let's make it as painless as possible. I'm going to teach you how to count your macros in a foolproof way (refer back to "Understand Your Macronutrients" on page 106). Then, after you complete the four-week program and enter Transition, you'll have the high fat and moderate protein dialed in, so you can simply track your net carbs going forward and define your personal limit.

I know this seems like a lot of work, but trust me: it's worth the investment. I failed keto until I took these steps and followed them carefully. Then I taught other women, such as Amy, how to do it too.

The key is to figure out the ketogenic ratio of your diet, so that you can reset your hormones. (And remember, this diet has been specifically designed for women's unique needs.) I'm going to walk you through the formula to calculate the ketogenic ratio over the next pages, but don't stress if this seems overly complicated at first. To make it easier, the specific food details in this chapter include sample meals!

Learning how to count macros is the best way to make sure your diet is activating ketones and improving your hormonal balance. You'll be shifting what you eat away from refined carbohydrates and toward healthy fats and certain proteins, which will increase the ketogenicity of your food—meaning that your body's ability to make ketones will improve because of the foods you eat.

Here's the basic formula for the ketogenic ratio:[12]

$$\text{Ketogenic Ratio} = \frac{\text{ketogenic factors}}{\text{anti-ketogenic factors}} = \frac{\text{fat (grams)}}{\text{carbs (grams) + protein (grams)}}$$

I want you to eat a ketogenic ratio of 2 ketogenic factors to 1 anti-ketogenic factor. That means you'll eat 2 grams of fat for every 1 gram of carbohydrate and protein combined. Most therapeutic applications of the ketogenic diet (such as those used for treatment of epilepsy) are more aggressive, asking for a ketogenic ratio of 4:1. That's tough to do if you want to eat a nutritionally sound food plan that includes vegetables; it requires a diet that is 90 percent fat and 10 percent a combination of protein and carbohydrates. I find that this type of keto diet may be too severe for many women.

Let's see what this looks like in real life. Say you are having scrambled eggs with spinach for breakfast. Here's how you calculate your ratio: 2 eggs contain about 12 grams of protein and 10 grams of fat. So you scramble 2 eggs in a pan with 1 tablespoon of olive oil (14 grams of fat) and add ¼ cup of spinach (contains less than ¼ gram of protein, less than ¼ gram of carbs, and less than ¼ gram of fiber — I'm going to call that a wash, or "0"). So the net, if you add these together, is 24 grams of fat in your scrambled eggs, with 12 grams of protein and carbs. That's 24:12, or the 2:1 ratio that we are seeking.

$$\textbf{Ketogenic Ratio} = \frac{\text{ketogenic factors}}{\text{anti-ketogenic factors}} \frac{24 \text{ (fat from the eggs and oil)}}{12 \text{ (protein from the eggs)}} = \frac{\text{fat (grams)}}{\text{carbs (grams)} + \text{protein (grams)}} \frac{2}{1}$$

Protein is more complicated. As you know, when the body gets more protein than it needs, the liver converts the extra protein into glucose in a process called gluconeogenesis. That's why the Gottfried Protocol is a *moderate protein* diet. (Read more details in the Notes.)[13]

This ratio will work if you follow an important rule: *you must not eat excess calories.* We all know that calories are not the only important part of a diet, but if you want to burn the fat you've stored at your waist, you need to follow the ketogenic ratio and make sure you don't eat more calories than you expend.[14] Fortunately, I can help you with that by specifying portion sizes with sample meals. I also provide more information on how to troubleshoot and avoid pitfalls in this chapter and the next.

You'll stick with this ketogenic ratio of 2:1 for three weeks, and then we will back off to a ketogenic ratio of 1:1 for the final week as we transition to a balanced low-carb food plan.

Read on for my goof-proof rules.

## THE DO'S AND DON'TS OF COUNTING YOUR MACROS

I'm going to make calculating the macronutrients (macros) of the ketogenic diet ridiculously simple. You have three main macros: fat, protein, and carbohydrates. We'll start with fat.

- **Do eat healthy fat.** Fat is the most calorie-dense of the macronutrients. Each gram of fat contains 9 calories, but not all sources of fat are created equal. There is still a lot of debate about the health benefits of saturated fat, so I want you to focus primarily on eating plant-based sources of fat, listed on page 117, and to limit saturated fat from animal sources.
- **Do eat moderate amounts of protein.** Each gram of protein contains 4 calories. You need to limit protein so that you stay in a ketogenic ratio of 2:1. See page 120 for healthy protein choices.
- **Do eat limited carbohydrates.** Each gram of carbohydrate has 4 calories, but once again, not all carbs are created equal. There is an optimal number of carbs that will allow you to lose weight, and we want to stay under it. This threshold is your *personal carb limit*. You can define it through trial and error, or you can take my advice (based on helping patients for the past thirty years), and stick to a limit of 20 to 25 grams of net carbs per day. (Not surprisingly, this is the same amount of net carbs that has been found to be the limit for healthy ketosis dating back to the 1970s.)[15] Most people who start a classic ketogenic diet restrict carbs (especially nonstarchy fibrous vegetables) too much, and the result is that their fiber count drops severely, from an average

of 28 grams to 6 grams per day.[16] Most keto programs use total carbs instead of net carbs, and usually aim for 20 to 35 grams per day. But that doesn't work for most women: we need fiber to support our hormones, especially estrogen and insulin, in order to keep them working best for weight loss. That's why it's important to learn how to track your net carbs each day.

- **Do limit net carbs to less than 25 grams per day.** Net carbs are the carbohydrates that are absorbed by the body. To calculate the net carbs in whole foods, subtract the grams of fiber from the total number of grams of carbs. I want you to limit processed foods, but even I eat them occasionally. (See examples in the Notes.)[17] NOTE: Your goal from Day 1 through Day 28 is to keep your net carbs below 25 grams per day. Practice this by recording your net carbs before Day 1 on your tracker, so you get the hang of it. To implement this strategy, plan ahead. Don't make the mistake of eating a meal and then checking the macros afterward — it's too late. Plan your menu a day in advance, and calculate the macros ahead of time. Say I plan to eat Avo Toast (see recipe on page 204). I'll toast one piece of keto bread (4 net carbs), mash one-third of an avocado (1 net carb), schmear it on the bread, and then drizzle 1 tablespoon of olive oil over top. The meal, a common breakfast for me, has a total of 5 net carbs and keeps me full for four to five hours.

- **Don't drink alcohol on Days 1 through 28.** I think of alcohol as liquid sugar. Women can't tolerate alcohol as well as men; they develop alcohol-related health problems at lower doses than men do. Alcohol interferes with the metabolism of estrogen and increases the risk of breast cancer.[18] And skipping your glass of wine may do more for your mental health than drinking it, according to a study published in 2019.[19] Alcohol has 7 calories per gram, so it's more calorie-dense than protein or carbs. Here's worse news: if you're carb intolerant, alcohol will kick you out of ketosis. *Alcohol blocks fat burning.* And that same quality that makes you feel more relaxed makes you more prone to second-guess your commitment and eat off the plan. If you are serious about weight loss, stay away from alcohol for at least three weeks. You can add it back during Transition if you must, and then you can see if you can stay in ketosis and continue to lose weight. If introducing alcohol causes a plateau in weight loss, back off from the sauce.

Here is a cheat sheet you can use to plan every meal during your first four weeks:

- Minimum fat: 20–40 grams
- Maximum protein: 10–20 grams
- Maximum net carbs (total carbs less total fiber): 7–10 grams, but less is preferable

If you are carb intolerant or insulin resistant, you may need to keep your carb limit even lower. (I cover this topic in the next chapter, where we talk about troubleshooting.) How do you know? Your waist is 35 inches or more as a woman, or 40 inches or more as a man. You are hungry most of the time because your appetite hormones are confused. Fat burning is close to impossible, and you are resistant to weight loss.

### From Dr. Sara's Case Files

"Thank you! I loved this program. It was a keto jumpstart for me. I've always wanted to try keto, and now I did. I lost 6 pounds [in the first ten days] on the program (and I didn't even work out because I am nursing an injury). Thank you!"
— *Amy, age forty-two and member of our online Gottfried Protocol Program*

## BECOME A BELIEVER (AND A TRACKER)

Let's say somebody came up to you and said, "I'll bet you $1,000,000 that you won't lose weight if you replace your rice crackers, granola bars, bagels, and pasta with bacon, avocados, cheese, and eggs."

Would you take the bet?

There was a time I wouldn't have, but now I would.

By the time you finish reading this chapter, I'm thinking you'll take that bet too. You now understand about restricting carbs the right way (that is, not dropping them too low and making sure they are the slow-burning type found in certain vegetables and a limited range of fruits). Putting this knowledge into action will allow your body to switch from burning sugar to burning fat as fuel. This produces ketones, which are especially supportive of brain function and stable energy for women over the age of thirty-five, when they start to hit early perimenopause.

I know this might feel like a lot of information to process, but I promise you, the hormone corrections and the pounds lost on the scale will make it worth this investment in your health. While attaining a healthy weight is important, it's not the only goal — we want to get you to a place of happier hormones, improved gut function, lower inflammation, restful sleep, more energy, and clearer thinking.

For the next four weeks, think of your food as a way for you to talk with your body. You're going to become fluent in the language of your hormones. The first word in this language is *fat*, the good kind. We're going to fight fire with fire or, more precisely, we're going to fight fat with fat.

**Preparation**
20–25 grams of net carbs and detoxification. Keep a ketogenic ratio of 2:1. Get your bowels moving so you can mobilize fat!

**Implementation**
20–25 grams net carbs per day, and add intermittent fasting (14/10 to 16/8). Continue a ketogenic ratio of 2:1.

**Transition**
Start to add net carbs slowly, 5 grams at a time, and heading toward a ketogenic ratio of 1:1 for the long term, or until you repeat the diet.

The Gottfried Protocol Timeline

# FROM MACROS TO MEALS: WHAT TO EAT ON THE GOTTFRIED PROTOCOL, AND WHY

Okay, now you've got the basics down — but how do they translate to your plate and what you eat each day?

## The Gottfried Protocol Loves Healthy Fat

Many of the hormones that we are trying to balance by means of the Gottfried Protocol are derived from cholesterol (a type of bodily fat found in all cells), so it makes sense that fat communicates best with your hormones. On the Gottfried Protocol, 60 to 70 percent of your diet will come from fat, mostly from plant-based sources, so it is critical to include fats with each meal. Eating more fat means you'll feel more satisfied (so you'll be more likely to stick with the program and not cheat). But keep in mind that fat is not "one size fits all." Some of my patients can have 2 tablespoons of coconut oil per day, and others hit a weight-loss plateau with that much saturated fat. Just as with carbs, when it comes to fat, you have to be the guinea pig and see what works best for you. Experiment with the following foods to expand your repertoire of healthy fats:

- **Avocado.** Sliced and placed on a salad, with lime juice drizzled over the top, or whipped as a base for creamy keto smoothies, avocados are a nutritional powerhouse. But before you go avo crazy, see How to Rock the Guac (page 124) for guidance on how much to enjoy.
- **Chocolate and cocoa.** You can have limited amounts of dark chocolate (90 percent cocoa solids or higher allowed), but consider going broader and using pure cocoa as a spice in savory dishes such as Mexican mole — delicious as a sauce for meat dishes.
- **Coconut.** Use 1 tablespoon per day of coconut oil during the twenty-eight-day program. See how you respond to it. In one study, coconut oil increased inflammation, as measured by blood

levels of something called endotoxin, whereas fish oil and cod liver oil decreased inflammation, and the effect of olive oil was neutral.[20] This is a great example of precision medicine — we need to understand what works best for you by finding the oils that reduce your inflammation.

- **Olive oil.** Use organic extra-virgin olive oil, and add it to virtually any dish. One of my mentors, Mark Houston, MD, recommends 5 tablespoons per day.
- **Nuts.** The best ketogenic varieties are macadamia nuts, walnuts, almonds, and pecans. Limit nuts to one serving, or 28 grams, per day. The heart-healthy and cancer-preventing benefits come at a dose of 12–30 grams per day, so take care not to eat too many.[21] For susceptible people, nuts can irritate the gut and trigger inflammation, owing to compounds like phytates and tannins, which can make them difficult to digest. You may notice gas, discomfort, or bloating after eating them. If you have an intolerance to nuts, skip them.
- **Seeds.** Sunflower, pumpkin, sesame, hemp, and flax — add these seeds to salads and other meals for a tasty crunch that is sure to satisfy some of those old habit memories.
- **Medium-chain triglyceride oil.** Take inspiration from Jen and add MCT to salads, smoothies, and vegetable dishes. Why? MCTs are a form of saturated fatty acid that is missing from the modern diet and has been shown to improve cholesterol profiles and to lower levels of fasting glucose and diastolic blood pressure.[22] Because it is efficiently used as energy, it is less likely to be stored as fat, so it can help support your weight-loss goals.[23] Specifically, taking MCT may help you eat less for the next forty-eight hours.[24] (More scientific details are in the Notes.)[25] Most women can tolerate ½ to 2 tablespoons per day. Too much may trigger diarrhea or make weight loss stall because of the caloric density. Personally, I aim for 1 tablespoon (20 grams) to 1.5 tablespoon (30 grams) per day in my shake or salad — 30 grams is the dose with the most positive proven effects.

One note of caution: As you start to plan your meals, th/portant thing to keep in mind is to avoid that deadliest combina... —high fat together with high carbs. This duo can increase inflammation, block insulin, and add to stored fat. Scientific studies show that a meal which includes saturated and trans fats, paired with refined carbohydrates, raises alarm bells in the body and significantly increases the risk of cardiovascular disease.[26] For the nerds like me who like to know more, this mechanism is described in greater detail in the Notes.[27]

### Your Daily Dose of Nuts

Nuts are brimming with vitamins, minerals, unsaturated fat, and antioxidants. They mostly consist of fat (about 50 to 75 percent), with a moderate amount of protein, making them an ideal keto food on the run. Research shows that people who eat their daily ounce of nuts (28 grams) minimize certain health risks: a 29 percent reduced risk of heart disease, a 24 percent lower likelihood of death from respiratory disease, and an 11 percent lower likelihood of death from cancer, according to the *New England Journal of Medicine*.[28]

Nuts are also dense in calories, so we need to get the dose right: high enough to reduce your risk of disease and support your transition to ketosis, but low enough that you aren't getting too many calories or irritating your gut.

Here is a rough guideline for that daily ounce:

- 30 pistachios
- 20 almonds
- 20 hazelnuts
- 15 macadamias
- 15 pecans
- 9 walnuts
- 2 tablespoons of pine nuts

## Eat Protein
## in Moderation

We've talked a lot about why you need to avoid excess protein; protein should make up 20 percent of your daily calories, but not all protein is created equal. Eating a factory-farmed beefsteak and its constituent inflammatory hormones, antibiotics, xenoestrogens, arachidonic acids, and omega-6 fats sends a fire-alarm message of inflammation to your hormones. Eating a grass-fed bison steak, with its clean protein and omega-3 fats, fuels your body and your hormones in a healthy way. In my opinion, the two meats shouldn't even be considered part of the same food group.

It is especially important to choose organic protein whenever possible because toxins that are rampant in conventionally raised meat confuse hormonal signaling, getting in the way of the clear message you're trying to send to your hormones during the Gottfried Protocol. Organic vegetables tend to have about 30 percent less pesticide residue[29] and reduce your exposure to antibiotic-resistant bacteria by a third, compared to conventional varieties. Good protein choices include the following items (in order of preference, starting with plants):

- Nuts (macadamia nuts, walnuts; see the list in "Your Daily Dose of Nuts").
- Seeds (pumpkin, flax, hemp).
- Eggs (from cage-free chickens).
- Wild-caught fish (varieties that are low in heavy metals, such as salmon, mackerel, sardines, trout).
- Shellfish (crab, mussels, oysters, scallops, shrimp).
- Free-range poultry (higher in omega-3 fats), preferably dark meat, with skin on.
- Organ meats (from free-range, grass-fed sources).
- Grass-fed beef and wild game (maximum of twice per week), including beef jerky with no added sugar.

- Pork (free of antibiotics and hormones, at a maximum of twice per week—avoid if weight increases)—choose pork chops, pork ribs, and pork rinds (I add chopped pork rinds to my salads as an alternative to croutons).

## Understand Carbs:
## The Body's False Energy

Carbohydrates are likely today's most confusing dietary element, trumping even cholesterol in the mixed-message department. Carbohydrates are a critical part of a diet that ensures optimal human function; however, for the past century, with the invention of factory food, carbohydrates all too often form the basis of an entire day's food plan. We've been drowning in carbohydrates, so our hormones are dismally out of balance. Their only recourse, when presented with another load of carbohydrates, is to tell the body to convert it to sugar and store it.

One reason for the carbohydrate confusion is that carbohydrates include a huge range of foods: everything from organic squash to angel food cake. And there are vast, contradictory messages about what to do with carbs. Ask a hundred nutritionists, and you'll get a wide spectrum of answers.

The Dietary Guidelines for Americans recommends that people consume 300 grams of carbs per day. I find this WAY off the mark for most people, particularly women over the age of thirty-five, who have waning levels of testosterone and growth hormone. Your optimal carb levels largely depend on the message you want to send to your hormones, your activity level, and whether you are male or female. Even the diet with the strongest scientific proof for preventing heart disease—the Mediterranean diet—recommends that 25–50 percent of daily calories come from carbohydrates. For an 1,800-calorie-per-day diet, that's 112 to 225 grams of carbohydrates, which is still too high. No wonder I started gaining weight on a Medi diet after age thirty-five!

The variance in carbohydrate recommendations doesn't mean they're all always wrong. If you're riding in the Tour de France and burning 5,000 calories each day, 300 grams will provide only about half of what you need. However, if you're like most Americans, living on highly processed simple carbohydrates laced with toxins for most of your life and eating more than you burn, you may need to reboot your daily carb consumption at an order of magnitude well below what the Dietary Guidelines recommend. After extensive research and experience with helping my patients work on weight loss, I find that a temporarily restrictive approach to carbohydrates, starting with 35–50 grams per day, and a maximum of 25 net carbs, is most effective.

What do 25 grams of net carbohydrate look like? When it comes to carbohydrate-dense grains, it's about the equivalent of a small pancake, ¾ of a cup of cooked pasta or rice, or most of a small bagel. My friend Jo, who loves carbs, asked me: did I mean individually or all together? Sorry, Jo: individually. Each of these options, too small to be satisfying, would complete your daily limit, so it's best to avoid them on the four-week program. Carbs also hide in sugars — ½ cup of sorbet or 1 cup of ice cream contains about 30 grams of carbs. (I know, right? We spent all those years opting for sorbet instead of ice cream to be healthier, yet as it turns out, sorbet has double the carbs!) You'll feel fuller from eating up to 30 grams of vegetables containing carbohydrates, which translates to about 8 cups of broccoli or cauliflower.

You're going to reduce carbohydrates over the short term, but increase fiber in order to beat your fat hormones and improve fat loss. Lowering net carbohydrates is the best method to reset your hormones — and we will do it by gently fasting and detoxifying, a topic we'll cover in the next chapter.

## Go Big on Veggies, Small on Fruit

The Protocol calls for myriad vegetables prepared with olive oil, but since we're limiting carbohydrates, particularly during the four-week program of the Gottfried Protocol, avoid starchy vegetables, including potato, corn, peas, winter squash, turnips, and beets. These can be reintroduced during the Transition phase.

For other vegetables, eat both raw and cooked varieties (cooking makes some nutrients more bioavailable, while destroying others), and prioritize vegetables that assist with detoxification, such as these:

- Leafy greens (arugula, kale, Swiss chard, collard greens, spinach, lettuces).
- Cauliflower, bok choy, broccoli, brussels sprouts, asparagus, bell peppers, onions, garlic, eggplant, cucumber, celery, summer squashes, zucchini, radishes, cabbages.
- Mushrooms.
- Limited starchy vegetables: jicama, pumpkin, winter squash during the Transition phase.

Sugars lurk in fruits in the form of fructose, so avoid most fruits during the four-week program. That said, certain fruits are lower in net carbs than others and are okay to include in small portions. (When you transition to eating more carbs during Transition, you can try adding small portions of low-glycemic fruits such as berries.) Gottfried Protocol–friendly fruits include these:

- Lemons.
- Limes.
- Olives.
- Tomatoes.
- Avocados. (Note that avocado is listed as a healthy fat, yet it's a fruit. See "How to Rock the Guac" so you don't get too much. The right amount for one serving is somewhere between ¼ and ½ of an avocado for most of my patients until they reach their weight goal.)

## Use Dairy with Care

Although dairy can be a significant source of healthy fat, there are reasons to use restraint. Some dairy products are high in natural lactose sugar. In randomized trials, increased dairy consumption is not associated with weight loss unless calories are decreased,[30] which usually occurs on a ketogenic diet because it is more satisfying and does result in weight loss. Calories matter, but hormones may matter more. Calories are less of a priority than getting your hormones back in balance. That means you can consume dairy, but not with abandon. Provided you are not dairy sensitive (that is, intolerant of casein, the main protein in milk) or lactose intolerant, and the dairy product is organic and sourced from grass-fed cows, you may include these healthy sources of fat:

- Butter.
- Hard cheeses.
- Other sugar-free and low-lactose dairy products.

Avoid high-lactose dairy products, including milk and ice cream.

## How to Rock the Guac

Before you whip up an avocado smoothie with a side of avocado slices dipped in guacamole, consider this: when I was trying keto for the first time to get back to an optimal weight, I overindulged in avocado, thinking it was a healthy fat that could be eaten without limit. Avocado is good for you, but only if eaten in the right amounts. Keep in mind that a whole avocado contains a significant amount of fat *and* carbs, so limit the amount to ¼ to ½ avocado per day. I'd rather have you eat a variety of diverse foods than use most of your daily carb allowance on avocado.

Nutrition information on the California Avocados website is based on the FDA-selected portion size for the food (⅓ of a medium avocado).[31] Since it's really easy to eat a whole avocado if you're not careful, this avocado nutrition table is adjusted for a whole medium-sized avocado, so you can see what you're getting if you do overindulge:

By the numbers, if you eat a whole avocado, you're consuming a third of your daily carb allowance, which doesn't leave much room for other nutritious carbohydrate foods. Be careful with avocado, at least until you've reached your healthy weight goal, which for most of my patients means achieving a BMI between 20 and 24.9.

### AVOCADO NUTRITION FACTS
*One medium avocado contains 3 servings*

| | |
|---|---|
| Total fat | 24 g |
| Saturated fat | 3 g |
| Trans fat | 0 g |
| Polyunsaturated fat | 3 g |
| Monounsaturated fat | 15 g |
| Cholesterol | 0 g |
| Sodium | 0 g |
| Total carbohydrate | 12 g |
| Dietary fiber | 9 g |
| Total sugar | 0 g |
| Added sugars | 0 g |
| Net carbohydrates | 3 g |
| Protein | 3 g |

## GET SPICY

It's been said that variety is the spice of life, and any nutrition plan will be more successful if it includes more palate-pleasing options. With that in mind, consider the following ways to add variety and flavor to your diet while still speaking the language of hormones:

- Dark chocolate (90 percent cocoa solids or higher).
- Unsweetened vinegars.
- Unsweetened coffee and tea.
- Unsweetened mustards.
- Spices: ginger, garlic, cayenne pepper, turmeric, cardamom, chili, fennel.
- Herbs: rosemary, parsley, cilantro, red clover, burdock root.

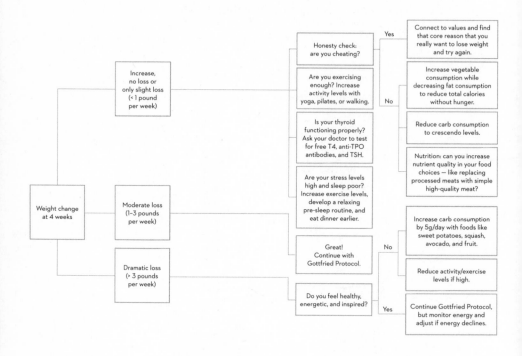

# SUGAR: THE WRONG HORMONAL MESSAGE

You know how fickle communication can be in a relationship, right? You say the right words twenty times in a row, and everything is flourishing. But then you slip up, say the wrong thing once, all hell breaks loose, and you destroy all the goodness. If the relationship has been solid for many years, it can handle the damage. However, if you slip up during those first few months of dating, it can spell the end.

Hormonal communication is no different. If you have a long history of supporting your hormones, a little sugar isn't going to hurt. But if you're like most women, and your metabolic hormones have been battered for decades by excess sugars, stress, and toxins, they need a good long stretch of virtuous communication. Think of the four-week Gottfried Protocol like those first delicate but thrilling months in a new relationship — don't send the wrong message.

With that in mind, here is the most destructive word in the language of the Gottfried Protocol: *sugar!*

I know I'm not the first to tell you sugar is bad, but when it comes to metabolic hormones, sugar is worse than you probably realize. Growth hormone is the ultimate metabolic hormone, and sugar is poison for it. Is it really that bad? Maybe even worse. Growth hormone improves insulin action,[32] and while clinical growth hormone deficiency is considered a rare condition, even minor alterations of growth hormone secretion are associated with metabolic and growth disorders.[33] When it comes to control of blood sugar, growth hormone does a job similar to that of cortisol and insulin,[34] but it does not cause the imbalances associated with these other two more famous hormones. Insulin and cortisol are aggressive and powerful, and they can overshoot easily, whereas growth hormone is more of a sensitive, New Age, likes-to-snuggle type. If you overload your system with sugar and stress, like so many of us do every day of our lives, cortisol and insulin dominate the dance floor while growth hormone plays wallflower.

This means you can't optimize growth hormone if you're indulging in double chocolate brownies, raising your blood sugar and inviting insulin to rise excessively. Dance with insulin for too long, and other hormones like growth hormone lose hope and become out of balance as your waist measurement expands. In healthy people, insulin blocks the release of growth hormone, and the hormone disruption may be even worse for people with obesity.[35] Eliminate added sugar from your diet, limit natural sugar, and, for the Preparation and Implementation phases of the Gottfried Protocol, avoid even seemingly healthy higher-sugar-content whole foods like bananas, grapes, and many other fruits. If you're insulin resistant, consider limiting these foods over the long term, until your insulin is repaired. Focus instead on healthy fats, anti-inflammatory proteins, and high-fiber foods like leafy greens and low-glycemic fruits (avocados, olives, coconut).

Sugar hides everywhere, so avoiding it isn't easy. During the four-week Gottfried Protocol, avoid sugar, even in its so-called healthy forms as listed here:

- Whole and refined grains and flour products.
- Added and natural sugars in food and beverages.
- Starchy vegetables like potatoes, corn, and winter squash. (Potatoes and squash can be added in limited amounts, such as 1–2 ounces, in the Transition phase.)
- Fruits other than those on the allowed list, unless factored into daily total carb consumption.
- All fruit juices.
- Legumes, including beans, lentils, and peanuts.
- Alcohol.

## WHAT DOES A MEAL WITH 70 PERCENT FAT LOOK LIKE?

Before we get into the meal possibilities, consider this: there are two ways to look at the question of what a meal with 70 percent fat looks like. First, what does it look like on the table, and second, what does it look like on you? The second part is maybe the more important, so I want to give you an objective data point from which to watch improvement happen: weight and waist circumference. And I'm going to start by giving you a lesson in how to properly collect these data points.

# INTEGRATION:
# GET YOUR DETOX ON

Why do the Preparation and Transition stages of the Gottfried Protocol include detoxification? Because detoxification and weight loss are inseparable, particularly for women. Detoxification is commonly the missing piece when it comes to creating a hormone-balancing ketogenic diet.

Fat is where the body squirrels away toxins (remember obesogens like BPA, the artificial chemicals that disrupt hormones and contribute to obesity?) when the natural detoxification system exceeds capacity. As fat is burned, the toxins are released into the bloodstream to be broken down and eliminated from the body; during rapid weight loss, the rate of toxins released from fat accelerates.[36] We need a way to keep removing the toxins, especially when more get released during weight loss. (I share more advanced detox strategies in Chapter 6 for people with stubborn weight gain.)

## The Three Phases of Detoxification

The body handles detoxification in three distinct phases: in phase one, the liver uses enzymes to break down harmful substances into a state that the body can handle; in phase two, the now-separate components of the compound are made soluble in water; and in phase three, they are eliminated from the body via urine, feces, or sweat. If you want to learn more about the phases of detox, refer to the Notes.[37] We will be focusing on phase three, so that you can promptly get rid of toxins released from fat.

To accomplish this goal, we'll use foods that bolster detox capacity. Despite being touted as a tool for weight loss, some food-detox programs have not demonstrated lasting results, but I'm going to show you how to do it correctly, so that you don't regain the weight.[38] That's why I've combined detoxification with ketogenic recommendations in a gentle, staged process. Look for opportunities to consume the following foods:

- **Clean, lean protein.** Without sufficient dietary protein, your liver cannot complete phase two detoxification, during which toxins are excreted.
- **Foods rich in fiber.** Among its many roles, fiber binds BPA and other toxins, helping your body excrete them. Smart high-fiber choices include avocados, olives, and nonstarchy vegetables. You can add supplemental fiber to shakes (see the Recipes). In the Transition phase of the Protocol, you can add back organic berries (no more than ¼ cup serving per day) and legumes (only in small portions, and none at all until the end of Implementation).
- **Foods rich in sulfur.** Detoxification pathways require this mineral, which is abundant in cruciferous veggies (broccoli and cauliflower among them, especially broccoli sprouts), onions, barnyard eggs, and garlic.
- **Healthy fat.** Inflammation forces your body to hoard toxins and contributes to nearly every disease on the planet. Wild-caught fish and flaxseed or chia seeds are among the many anti-inflammatory fatty foods that help your body detoxify.
- **Filtered water.** Among its many duties, water helps eliminate toxins and boosts cellular energy, tissue structure, and nutrient processing. Choose filtered water (use a simple carbon filter or get more fancy with reverse osmosis) so you're not flooding your body with more pollutants, like the heavy metals and other potentially harmful substances common in tap water. Drink more than you did before starting the diet because we are here to *change things* in your body. Further, dehydration is one of the two most common complications of the ketogenic diet (the other is gastrointestinal upset) during the first month.[39] You should hydrate like an athlete, particularly during the first two to three weeks. Increased hydration will support detoxification and reduce the issues known to be associated with ketogenic diets and other weight-loss programs, while giving you the best chance of sustaining the benefits of the program over time. Add electrolytes to your

water (see my favorite keto-friendly brands in the Resources). Aim for 60 or more ounces per day of filtered water, which will make you get up to urinate once an hour.

## ADJUST FOR YOUR METABOLOTYPE

As mentioned in Chapter 4, whether you have an apple or pear metabolotype, there is a way to personalize the Gottfried Protocol for you. Women with an apple metabolotype need more detoxification, fewer carbs (at least temporarily, for four weeks), and deeper ketosis (by which you produce significant amounts of ketones, measured as greater than 1.0 mmol/L in the blood). (In the next chapter, you will learn how to check for ketosis.) Be sure to follow the basic guidelines for detoxification in this chapter as well as the more advanced strategies described in Chapter 6. Aim for 20 grams or fewer net carbs per day to start. Add intermittent fasting, with the goal of a fourteen-hour overnight fast starting twice per week.

Pears can get away with lighter ketosis (in which the body is producing ketones from burning fat in smaller quantities, measured at 0.5–1.0 mmol/L in the blood) but respond well to intermittent fasting. Try consuming 25 or fewer net carbs per day, and add intermittent fasting every night for fourteen hours. This is particularly helpful for women over forty who are in perimenopause or menopause and feel like all their fat migrated to their hips and butt.

This customization, together with the troubleshooting suggestions and plateau busters in the next chapter, provide powerful tools to help you progress toward wellness.

## A SAMPLE DAY ON
## THE GOTTFRIED PROTOCOL

Making more food at home will give you the greatest success with weight loss. Eating out is associated with diabetes and weight gain,[40] so do your best to curb the dine-in or take-out habit and replace it with nutritious homemade meals. Not a cook? No need to stress. I will show you how to become a master of meal assembly.

On Day 1, you'll eat 70 percent fat and limit your carbs to a huge salad. In the next two chapters, we'll get into each phase of the Gottfried Protocol in detail, but for now, here are some examples of what meals might look like at the breakfast table, at both a sit-down lunch and a grab-and-go quick one, and at dinner, including an out-on-the-town evening of fine dining and a home-cooked meal.

**Breakfast**

*Sit down:* Keto granola with coconut milk (2 net carbs total, in grams).

*On the run:* Avocado on keto toast (6 net carbs). (See recipe for Avo Toast, page 204.)

**Lunch**

*Home cooked:* 6 ounces brussels sprouts sautéed with 3 ounces grass-fed brisket, and a small side salad with detoxifying greens such as watercress and broccoli sprouts.

*On the run:* By the start of Implementation, you'll have a soup to grab from the freezer. When you're starting the Protocol, try to avoid fast food, but if you have no other option, here are a few suggestions. Get a salad with guacamole and your choice of protein from Chipotle Mexican Grill (they have a keto salad listed under their lifestyle bowls — but avoid tortillas, tortilla chips, and corn). Or get a burger wrapped in lettuce and skip the french fries.

**Dinner**

*Home cooked:* 6 ounces mashed cauliflower with turkey meatballs and truffle oil, plus a side salad.

*On the town:* A wide range of meals can fit the plan if you tiptoe around the carbs and low-quality fats. Ask for salad, a side of avocado, or steamed nonstarchy vegetables (I usually order a "double") as a substitute for the carbs. Ask for a side of olive oil and fresh lemon for salad dressing. Avoid dessert, sauces, and glazes, and always ask if sugar is used in the preparation of a dish.

See Chapter 9 for more than sixty Gottfried Protocol recipes, along with Seven-Day Meal Plans for a variety of dietary preferences, including vegetarian and vegan. See Resources for product recommendations.

## Dr. Sara's Secret Keto Weapon: Soups

Soups add diversity, comfort, and convenient nutrition to a ketogenic diet. They make great leftovers for a meal the next day or a grab-and-go lunch pulled from the freezer. When you are wringing your hands because you're tired and can't think of what to eat for dinner, you'll be happy that you made a batch of Chicken-Ginger Soup, Tofu Masala Soup, Creamy Goddess Greens Soup, or a simple vegetable soup. Just pull a jar out and defrost it.

My other favorites are a keto version of the hearty Greek meal-in-a-bowl called Avgolemono (chicken soup with lemon and riced cauliflower), chicken zoodle soup, and in the summer, Gazpacho — mine is heavy on the cucumbers and avocado. You'll find these recipes and more in Chapter 9, along with time-saving tips and suggested products that will make meal prep manageable and the results delicious.

I cook my soup bases on Sunday, and stock the refrigerator and freezer for the week. Get creative with nonstarchy vegetables in a base of bone broth or vegetable broth. When you reheat the base, add fish, shellfish, meat, more vegetables, and extra-virgin olive oil.

## FINAL SENDOFF:
## IT'S ONLY FOUR WEEKS!

At this point, you may be thinking that it's all too much—you just want to eat a cupcake and call it a day. Don't put off your health and hormones for another minute. Yes, this plan is asking you to change the way you eat. And yes, you will need a high level of precision to hit the right ketogenic ratio. Don't let this worry you. Remember: we are talking about only four weeks, and I'm providing you with all of the support you need for success.

Before you panic and reminisce about all of the food habit memories you can't enjoy anymore, I have good news: I provide a hormone-benefiting version of each of these carb-laden treats. We will swap the chips for keto crackers, lose the croissant but enjoy keto bread with nut butter, and swap pasta for shirataki noodles (made from Japanese konjac root, with zero net carbs). Over the past few years, I've found the swaps that satisfy my cravings without telling my hormones to nosedive, and I'm so excited to share them with you.

Now you understand that if your hormones aren't balanced, no amount of dieting or exercise will work. And now you know what to do to fix it. Following the steps and the macros that we cover in this chapter and applying it to your next meal is your first big leap into getting your hormones back on track, by getting your food on board. Balanced hormones + less hunger = weight loss. Let's do this!

## *Highlights*

▶ Get your food to send the right information to your hormones.
▶ Don't let habit memories bring you down. Replace unhealthy habit memories with keto swaps that will form new, health-supporting habit memories (see Resources for more ideas).
▶ Familiarize yourself with the three steps — understand the hormone-food connection, be the guinea pig, and count your macros — before you begin Day 1.

► Remember: we are pulsing to a ketogenic ratio of 2:1 (fats in proportion to protein plus carbs, all in grams) for four weeks, and then we will back off to a ketogenic ratio of 1:1.

I've included all of the resources you need for success, including troubleshooting tips, recipes, meal plans, and product recommendations.

# 6

---

# DETOXING, CIRCADIAN FASTING, AND TROUBLESHOOTING

Now that you understand how most diets can make women crash hormonally, and you are armed with macronutrient targets and the 2:1 ketogenic ratio, we are ready to fine-tune your fat loss. Together we will find your sweet spot, so you'll feel satiated as your hormones settle into place, the belly fat shrinks, and you lose weight. This creates the orchestra that plays the music of life to your 60 to 90 trillion cells. In this chapter, I'll share with you the lessons I learned the hard way so that you'll be spared the trial and error in accelerating hormone balance. Armed with the tips and tricks in this chapter, you can leapfrog into trial and success.

Some of my patients are like Lara, who lost 5 pounds in the first five days and entered ketosis, firmly crossing the line from "overweight" (BMI 25–30) to "normal" (BMI less than 25.0) *Five days!* She went on to lose another 4 pounds by the end of week two, but then hit a plateau. I'll show you what worked for Lara, and what can work for you if you encounter resistance to weight loss—a phenomenon that is unfortunately very common for women over thirty-five. But with science-backed solutions, it can be overcome.

Lara's experience is very common on the Gottfried Protocol.

When you reduce carbohydrates, you initially lose weight fast because carbohydrates drag water with them. But then weight loss may slow down as the body gets adjusted to burning fat. This is known as becoming keto-adapted, or fat-adapted. Lara is 5 feet, 8 inches tall and began the program at 165 pounds, giving her a BMI of 25.1 kg/m² (mildly overweight). Our first goal for Lara was to lose 5 pounds of mostly fat mass. She accomplished that goal. Ultimately, her goal is to weigh 145 pounds, with a healthy BMI of 22. You'll hear more about her progress with busting her plateau and the "what next?" answers that really help when you need to keep burning fat despite the slowdown.

Here are the questions we'll answer:

- What reasonable weight-loss goals can you achieve and sustain with the Gottfried Protocol?
- Is detoxification proceeding successfully?
- How do you accelerate hormonal repair by layering in circadian-based intermittent fasting?
- What are the top seven pitfalls to avoid?

Most of all, keep in mind one of my mottos: imperfect action trumps perfect inaction (something I paraphrased from President Harry Truman). You can start late, start over, try and fail, and ultimately try and succeed. All those micro decisions I'm asking you to make will add up to a major transformation. That's been my own experience in developing and refining the Gottfried Protocol. Don't aim for perfection — it is the enemy of good. I only ask that you stay on the path and be kind to yourself. Hang in there long enough to let your hormone, gut, and brain circuits catch up.

## SET REALISTIC GOALS

As you enter nutritional ketosis, set small goals. I like to begin with 5 pounds of weight loss, with preserved muscle mass. The best way to track this is by measuring your weight daily after your morning bowel movement (if you are not having a bowel movement every morning, see the detox troubleshooting guide later in the chapter). Measure your waist at belly-button level weekly, using the technique described in the last chapter. If you are losing fat and preserving muscle mass, your weight will decline and your waist circumference will decrease. (See the Notes for more advanced techniques.)

What's a reasonable amount of weight loss? There are many factors to consider: age, resting metabolic rate (how fast or slow you burn calories), baseline hormones, activity level, stress, and how much weight you have to lose to get to your goal BMI.

My recommendation is to aim ultimately for a BMI of 18.5 to 24.9, but to break it down into steps. If your BMI is above 24.9, begin with the goal of losing 5 percent of your weight or 5 pounds of mostly fat. Why? It's a manageable goal that has been shown to have a beneficial effect on health, particularly for those with polycystic ovary syndrome (PCOS) — the most common type of metabolic disturbance that women experience.

Lara, who began the Gottfried Protocol at 165 pounds, had lost 5 pounds by Day 5. She lost 5 percent of her weight (8.25 pounds) by Day 12 of the Protocol. By Day 22, she was down 10 pounds, with a total weight of 155 pounds. One month later, she weighed 150 pounds.

Like Lara, you probably gained weight gradually. The average woman gains 2 pounds per year from age sixteen to age thirty-six.[1] Scientists have shown that this weight gain is subtle, representing as little as 20 extra calories per day, likely combined with wayward activity of hormones like cortisol and insulin. That means we need to lose the pounds gradually too, for this important reason: rapid weight loss is rarely sustainable. Go slow. I know you're desperate to lose weight — I've been there too. But your palate, your brain circuits (including your set point, the way your brain regulates body fat within a narrow range, similar to a thermostat, based on food intake and exercise), your gut (from the taste receptors in your mouth to the stretch receptors in your stomach), and your hormones have been hijacked by years, if not decades, of adulterated food and an environment that promotes fat storage (known as an obesogenic environment). We can fix this problem. If you follow my guidelines, you'll have to complete this process only once.

To improve your outcome, I recommend that you perform the Gottfried Protocol with a friend. We know that accountability can improve results. When I succeeded in my third attempt at keto, I texted my weight every morning to a friend, and she did the same. We kept each other motivated and engaged through daily connection and our affirming words of support!

# Q&A WITH DR. SARA

**Q:** *Can I have a cheat day?*

**A:** No. Keto isn't like diets that allow for a cheat day. You must eat at least a 2:1 ketogenic ratio to get the hormonal benefits of a ketogenic diet. Furthermore, most of my patients find it easier to follow a strict diet, 100 percent of the time, rather than 95 or 98 percent. I've been there myself, plus science backs up this principle. Dairy is a common ingredient in cheat meals, and it can kick you out of ketosis by raising insulin (see the next chapter, on food intolerances). One day of sugar and flour, and the sugar cravings and morphine-like substances derived from gluten and casein (very sedating and addictive opioids called gluteomorphins and caseomorphins) are back in charge. Don't do it. Four weeks of strict, 100 percent adherence will get you the best results.

## KEEP MEASURING

In addition to tracking your macronutrients (fat, protein, total carbs, net carbs), daily weight, and weekly waist circumference, we will layer in measuring ketones. Here's something I constantly communicate to my patients: what you measure improves. You direct your intentions and attention toward measurement, and it will help you reach your goal.

Many people take two to seven days to enter ketosis after starting my Protocol. I highly recommend testing yourself for ketones, an important metric, because if weight loss stalls, you will have the data to pinpoint why.

Back in the days of the Atkins diet, people would pee on a test strip to check for ketones in the urine. This can work initially, but once you become keto-adapted, you are less likely to continue spilling ketones into your urine. I recommend a blood ketone monitor that measures beta-hydroxybutyrate; it may be the most important ketone when you're in ketosis and has many benefits in terms of improving metabolism. When you are firmly in ketosis during Implementation, your blood ketones should measure 0.5 to 3.0 millimolar (mmol/L). A blood ketone level that is less than 0.5 mmol/L indicates that the body is not in ketosis.

No other diet has a metric that tells you if you're doing it effectively. Isn't that cool? The best way to check your ketones and glucose levels is to do so at the same time each day (see Resources for devices that measure both). For most busy women, that's first thing in the morning, after measuring your weight. I measure while drinking a large glass of filtered water since we all tend to wake up dehydrated, particularly when in ketosis. Getting into the testing habit will make the final week, Transition, easier, as you start to test for your personal carbohydrate limit. Additionally, I like to check glucose two hours after I eat (also called postprandial or meal glucose), as that can better identify a different type of problem with insulin than fasting glucose alone can.

# Q&A WITH DR. SARA

**Q:** *My ketones were 0.3 mmol/L on Day 1, then 0.7 mmol/L on Day 3. Then I started my period, and now my ketones are 0.4 mmol/L on Day 7. Is this normal?*

**A:** This is an example of why you might need a food log, in which you track your weight and ketones each morning, along with every food and drink that you consume. In the same log, you can track your macronutrients and net carbs. I urge my patients to keep a log as an online spreadsheet and to share it with me for troubleshooting, as needed. The best way to unravel why you fell out of ketosis is to review your log and take note of patterns. Some of my patients crave more carbohydrates before their period and pop out of ketosis when they consume more than 20 to 25 net carbs per day. Similarly, we can use the log to identify the foods that help you enter a deeper state of ketosis.

## TRACK YOUR GLUCOSE KETONE INDEX (GKI)

A biomarker is a measure that tells you if something in particular is happening in your body. GKI is a biomarker that can help you track your progress on the Gottfried Protocol—it's one of the best indicators of your metabolic state. GKI shows the relationship between your ketone levels and your glucose levels, measured by a simple formula: dividing your blood glucose level (must be in the units mmol/L) and your blood ketone level (mmol/L).

Originally developed as way of tracking progress with cancer treatment,[2] measuring GKI can help us track whether both variables —glucose and ketones—are collectively heading in the right direction. In medicine, this measure is also used for patients with diabetes, obesity, Alzheimer's disease, Parkinson's disease, epilepsy, insulin resistance, and traumatic brain injury. For weight loss, the GKI is the most helpful single biomarker that I use to track a patient's success with the Gottfried Protocol — it is far more helpful than tracking glucose and ketones independently, since daily life, stress, activity, and nutrition may interfere with individual measurements. We are looking for trends.

Generally, I recommend a GKI of 1–3 to address problems with obesity, insulin resistance, circadian health, sleep, and weight loss. A GKI of 3–6 is still helpful for repairing insulin block, and a GKI of 6–9 still has weight-loss benefits.

### How to Calculate Your GKI

[Glucose (mg/dL)/18]/ketone (mmol/L)

If you are outside the United States, use this calculation, which is more direct: glucose (mmol/L)/ketone (mmol/L).

If you are in the United States, you need to use a correction of 18.0 to convert the glucose reading from mg/dL to mmol/L units.

## KEEP UP THE DETOXIFICATION

To deepen and accelerate the balancing of hormones that occurs with the ketogenic diet, continue the detoxification. We want to keep refreshing your liver detoxification pathways so that you can clear the toxins released as you burn more fat. Here are many practical ideas to assist you.

### Detox and Food

- Eat more cruciferous vegetables. You use the very same receptor on cells for environmental toxins that you use for cruciferous vegetables, so you can crowd out the toxins by eating them.[3]
- Eat sulforaphane daily. This nutrient is found in the highest concentrations in cruciferous vegetables (broccoli, brussels

sprouts, cabbage, cauliflower, kale, radishes). It helps multiple
liver detox pathways and has been found to improve leaky gut.

- Keep eating green leafy vegetables, zucchini, cucumber, and
eggplant. Vegetables trigger a cleanup of the immune system.
Most of my patients can eat these vegetables without limit
and do not need to bother counting them; the same finding
is reported by other keto researchers.[4] However, you must
continue counting your other macronutrients, particularly those
vegetables not listed here, protein, and fats.

- Track all macros. My hope is that you will completely
eliminate processed foods, but if not, count those macros
religiously as well.

- Avoid toxins whenever possible, particularly genetically
modified foods and wine (which you aren't drinking during
the four-week cycle anyway); they contain glyphosate, the
most common herbicide.[5] Glyphosate inhibits growth hormone
and will work against your fat-loss goals. Read more in the
Notes about a supplement that may help repair the gut after
glyphosate exposure.[6]

- Avoid *obesogens,* chemicals that can disrupt your body's
hormones and make you fat. These man-made environmental
chemicals can cause weight to increase.[7] Obesogens include
some medications (for example, selective serotonin reuptake
inhibitors, or SSRIs), pesticides, and xenobiotics like bisphenol
A (BPA), a known obesogen. Unfortunately, it's tough to
completely avoid these chemicals. Endocrine disruptors exist
in plastic bottles, printed receipts, metal food cans, detergents,
foods, toys, and skin care products. One animal study found that
BPA suppresses growth hormone and release.[8] It disrupts the
microbiome, the environment of gut bacteria that is crucial to
our health, influencing how we absorb nutrients and experience
cravings and even moods.[9] One healthy option is to eat more
probiotic food and consider taking probiotics, which may help

decrease the effects of BPA and other toxins; this has been shown to be the case in studies of animals.[10]

- Consider your home, work, and even vacation environments more broadly. Are any obesogenic, meaning they promote weight gain and are not conducive to weight loss? (See the following "Q&A with Dr. Sara.")

- Eat these for the best source of support for the liver: cruciferous vegetables (notice the theme), shiitake mushrooms, turmeric, and rosemary. Berries provide important nutrients to support liver function too, but you will need to make sure that when eating them in the first four weeks of the Gottfried Protocol, you follow the 2:1 ketogenic ratio with your macros. Most of my patients wait to eat berries until Day 29, during Transition. That is when we'll look more closely at gradually increasing carb intake and seeing how you respond.

# Q&A WITH DR. SARA

**Q:** *What actions can I take to detoxify obesogenic environments?*

**A:** You don't just have to eliminate toxins in your food; living or working in a toxic environment can be just as harmful for your health and your waistline. What do I mean by a toxic environment? It can come in many forms. Maybe it's an office culture that encourages ordering take-out rather than bringing in your own healthy lunch. Or spending time with loved ones who prefer to watch TV while consuming a bag of tempting, carb-loaded snacks. Come up with creative ways to circumvent these potential pitfalls, and reclaim your space. For example, take a walk at lunch or after dinner, or keep fresh celery sticks handy in the fridge for when you crave some "crunch."

## Detox and Bowel Movements

- Be sure you are completely evacuating your bowels at least once or twice per day. That means you don't feel like there's still any stool that's stuck in your colon or rectum.
- Eat and drink the right stuff. To keep your gut moving, you will require sufficient hydration, high-fiber vegetables, and possibly a magnesium supplement.
  - Drink plenty of filtered water, at least half of your body weight (measured in pounds) in ounces. So, for Lara at 165 pounds, that's 77.5 ounces of filtered water each day. By the way, her weight loss improved when she increased to 90. She adds keto-friendly (no sugar) electrolytes.
  - Eat high-fiber vegetables plus 25 grams of lettuce daily (see Recipes for a list of ideas, from romaine to red leaf).
  - Add 1–2 tablespoons of ground flaxseed to a shake bowl (see Recipes) or shake.
  - Include 1–2 tablespoons of MCT oil with each meal.
  - Consider taking a magnesium supplement. More than half of US adults are low in magnesium, a condition that can block many hormone pathways and harm your health.[11] I aim to get my Gottfried Protocol patients to 800 milligrams per day, but you can find the right dose for you by starting at 200–300 milligrams and slowly increasing the amount. Note that magnesium supplements may interact with certain medicines, and may not be appropriate for those with diabetes, intestinal disease, heart disease, or kidney disease. Please speak with your health care provider if you are taking medicines or have one of these conditions.

# Q&A WITH DR. SARA

**Q:** *I am following all of your recommendations, but I'm still not having a bowel movement every day. What else can I do?*

**A:** A daily bowel movement is healthy and detoxifying. I have a lot of patients with constipation, and it can take a while to normalize the transit time of food as it travels through your gut. I think of this list of actions — drinking more filtered water, getting your nonstarchy veggies, adding flaxseed and MCT to your meals, and taking magnesium — as the basics. Just like a shampoo for your hair, you want to keep up a consistent pattern of lather, rinse, repeat. Some of my patients improve their transit time by adding the Ayurvedic herb triphala, either in powder form (mixed with water) or as a capsule, to their list of supplements. Other common causes of constipation include toxic stress, thyroid problems, and missing micronutrients. If you get up to 800 milligrams of magnesium, plus you are doing all of the other activities, I recommend that you consult with a functional medicine clinician to further evaluate your gut.[12]

## Detox and Sweating

- Exercise to the point of sweating, which will help you excrete toxins. I am obsessed with this combination: two-thirds lifting with heavy weights, even at home, and one-third cardio. However, exercise tends to make me ravenously hungry, so I use a kitchen scale to measure my food. Exercise moves your lymphatics, which helps with detoxification. Overall, the goal is sweat.
- Another way to sweat is to soak in a hot bath with Epsom salts. Begin an hour or more before you expect to fall asleep. Let's just say I order Epsom salts by the 32-pound bucket, and that amount will carry you through the Gottfried Protocol. I add 4

cups of Epsom salts, about 1–2 cups of baking soda, a few drops of at least two essential oils (a mix, on repeat, is spruce and frankincense) and then I soak in the hottest water I can tolerate for 20 minutes or more. (My dose of Epsom salts has increased since I wrote about them in *The Hormone Reset Diet.*) Then I lie in bed over a towel while I continue sweating, and I read a favorite book. This is another way to restore magnesium, and it's delightfully relaxing before sleep. Think of it as a hormone-balancing alternative to a cocktail — one that actually helps you relax while improving your sleep.

- Try a sauna. I can't say enough about its benefits. It's another way to sweat without the exercise and the increase in appetite that can result. In today's world, where so many toxins seem unavoidable, a sauna is one way of removing them. Installing a sauna in your home is a sound investment — you'll pay for it when you sell your house, and it will keep your brain and body clear of certain toxins. The data on sauna use for detoxification support contain gaps, but the findings are sufficient to get my nod of approval.[13]
- Explore additional supplements to support the liver:
  - N-acetyl cysteine (NAC) helps protect the liver from damage and may regulate female hormones.[14] For some women with PCOS, it may improve insulin levels,[15] though not for all.[16] Dose: 600 milligrams twice per day.
  - Milk thistle has been shown to decrease liver inflammation and lower blood glucose in diabetic patients.[17] Dose: 140 milligrams three times daily for forty-five days.
  - Turmeric extract has been shown to protect against liver injury, help patients with fatty liver, improve total and low-density cholesterol, and possibly reduce blood glucose and body mass index (BMI).[18] Dose: 500 milligrams per day.

## Other Lifestyle Changes

- Become a super sleeper. Quality sleep is important for detoxification as well the production of growth hormone and testosterone. Your body produces growth hormone during deep sleep, so aim for seven to eight and a half hours of total sleep each night, and, if you track it, about 90 to 120 minutes of deep sleep. Develop a bedtime ritual that includes removing screens for the last hour, and avoid eating at least three hours before bedtime.

- Rise above toxic stress. We are all so tense and inflamed. My method to unwind and reset is yoga, including daily meditation. I write about stress relief in all of my books because stress hormones tend to block fat loss, and it will serve you well to find effective ways to become stress resilient. No method is good or bad or better; the key is to find what's right for you. I suggest trying yoga or a meditation app, like Calm or Headspace or Ten Percent Happier. For certain people, yoga or meditation or mindfulness feels alien or they cannot sit still. That's okay. Try it anyway. I think of yoga as a fundamental key to reset your body's endocrinology, whereby you replace negative hormones with more positive ones. Less cortisol and insulin, more testosterone, oxytocin, and growth hormone.

# Q&A WITH DR. SARA

**Q:** *I've been stressed and have started craving and eating more carbs again. What can I do?*

**A:** We've all been there. I call it carb creep. When you start to eat excess carbohydrates (that is, over your limit), you may also notice fluid retention, and the scale can climb because of more water weight. I see this commonly in patients who eat take-out food or eat out at restaurants, where carbs are often hidden in the food. Weight can spiral up over time, and you can gain 5 pounds or more until you identify and address the problem. Don't let that happen.

Here's are the questions that I ask my patients: Are you tracking every food and drink you consume? Are you weighing yourself every morning and measuring your ketones and GKI? What you measure improves. Are you calculating net carbs for every meal, before you eat it? Are you covering the basics by drinking plenty of filtered water, avoiding sugar and alcohol, and eating lightly steamed non-starchy vegetables? Are you making signature meals and soups? (See Recipes.) Are you moving, pooping, and sleeping? Do you have an accountability partner to whom you text or email your daily progress and with whom you troubleshoot challenges? On a deeper level, take an abdominal breath, and make a list of things you can do besides eat carbs when you feel stressed. Here's my list: text a friend, call one of my sisters, go for a walk, hop on the exercise bike, swing a kettlebell twelve times, do ten burpees, talk to my husband, breathe deeply or meditate for 5 minutes, drink a glass of filtered water, read a book, or take a nap.

If you notice carb creep, nip it in the bud right away by recommitting to the basics of the Gottfried Protocol.

# CIRCADIAN-BASED INTERMITTENT FASTING: AN EASY, HEALTHY HABIT

I tried keto twice for fat loss before I got it to work for my hormones. As I look back on what I did wrong, it all looked right from the outside. I was eating macros in the desired range: 70/20/10. I entered ketosis. But the first time, I ate too much fat — probably too many saturated fat calories for me (butter in my coffee, liberal amounts of bacon and cheese in my diet). The second time, I didn't eat enough vegetables, and my gut microbes suffered. I didn't mop up the toxins first. I was eating breakfast, lunch, and dinner, plus snacks in between. Oh, and I didn't stop drinking alcohol — that's a longer story, but I've got several hacks for you in this chapter if you can't imagine life without your nightly glass of wine!

The third round of ketosis worked: I lost 20 pounds of mostly fat. What was different: circadian-based intermittent fasting, a focus on detoxification, and eating in a way that honors female hormones, including giving up alcohol. Leveraging this combination of factors, the Gottfried Protocol is a weight-loss accelerator.

Intermittent fasting is a back door to ketosis, because most people produce ketones after sixteen or so hours of fasting. When you eat within a window that leverages circadian rhythm, your body will be more aligned with the release of nearly every hormone that you produce. This means that if you start eating several hours after the sun rises (ideally after a fasted workout) and stop eating a few hours before the sun sets, you will be working with and not against how the human body, male and female, evolved to eat—with extended periods of metabolic rest. Now we work longer days and use artificial light at night, so our eating patterns less and less resemble the way they evolved. The worst-case scenario for your metabolic hormones is for you to eat a big meal and then go to bed, yet that's what most people do. For the benefit of your hormones, you need to be in a state of fasting every night when you go to bed.

Of all the programs I have utilized with thousands of patients in my clinic over twenty-five years, time-restricted eating is the easiest behavioral modification to encourage weight loss, especially for women. In a 2019 University of Illinois at Chicago study, obese adults lost about 3 percent of their body mass by adhering to a 16:8 diet.[19] The plan was simple: the participants limited their food intake to only eight hours per day. And they fasted for the other sixteen.

When you combine circadian-based intermittent fasting with eating ketogenic food, you produce more ketones faster, which can aid weight loss. You can get the Gottfried Protocol benefits without hunger or deprivation by closing your kitchen after dinner, thereby creating an approximate fourteen-to-sixteen-hour window during which you shift into fat-burning, insulin-and-growth-hormone-optimizing mode. (Don't worry: most of that fasting will occur while you sleep.)

Your effort will be rewarded with optimal levels of insulin and growth hormone (and other hormones), fat loss, increased energy and stamina, and other health benefits. Achieving *mild* ketosis through a sixteen-hour overnight fast increases mental acuity, lowers blood sugar, resets insulin block, triggers autophagy (clearing out of damaged cells), repairs DNA, and regulates mTOR (the gene involved in your health span, or healthy life span).

## The Science of Circadian-Based Intermittent Fasting

Studies of humans and animals indicate that circadian-based intermittent fasting has the following benefits:

- Reverses weight gain.[20]
- Restores the normal expression of genes involved in diet-induced obesity, especially in models of postmenopausal obesity.[21]
- Improves blood sugar (heals insulin block).[22]
- Lowers cardiometabolic risk.[23]
- Reduces risk of breast cancer and other cancers.[24]
- Markedly reduces aging.[25]
- Turns white fat into more metabolically favorable brown fat, so that you burn more calories.[26]
- Reshapes gut microbiota in favor of obesity-protective bacteria (for example, *Oscillibacter, Ruminococcaceae*), and contributes to microbiota diversity, a universal hallmark of health.[27]
- Improves the metabolic consequences of a disrupted circadian clock.[28]
- May help the brain ward off neurodegenerative diseases like Alzheimer's, other forms of dementia, and Parkinson's, while improving mood and memory.[29]

And intermittent fasting does all of this without curbing calories or requiring a specific dietary strategy![30]

Some of you may succeed with a rapid dive into intermittent fasting. I advise most of my female patients to ease into it, however, since it can be stressful for the body, and we don't want to raise cortisol levels by adding more stress. Here's how to do it.

# HOW TO EASE INTO INTERMITTENT FASTING

1.  Start with tracking your normal food pattern, and introduce time-restricted eating with an overnight fast of twelve to fourteen hours on nonconsecutive days—and a corresponding eating window of twelve to ten hours, respectively—with *adaptive exercise only* (Pilates, yoga, walking) on those days. You can do this on Day 1 or begin at any time during the four-week Protocol. The sooner you start, the sooner you will see more hormonal benefits.

2.  During this gradual ramping up, eat more of your carbs at breakfast in the morning, if possible, because that is when we are more insulin sensitive and can burn the carbohydrates as fuel. Eat low carb at dinner—this is a great time to eat fish or take omega-3 supplements to help you feel satisfied longer. Keep within your total carb and net carb limits each day.

3.  Fast for three or more hours before bedtime, as this is the most insulin-resistant time of day.

4.  Consume only healthy noncaloric drinks in the morning. Black coffee or tea first thing are okay and do not break your fast. There is debate as to whether calories, such as a tablespoon of cream in your coffee, break the fast. The most conservative approach is to stick to water, black coffee, or green tea, with nothing added.

5.  Break your fast in the morning with nutrient-dense food. This is when I eat keto Avo Toast or a green smoothie packed with vegetables, nuts, and seeds.

6.  Continue to follow the Gottfried Protocol dietary recommendations from the previous chapter: Eat whole, minimally processed foods prepared at home whenever possible. Avoid added sugar, refined flour, and trans fats. Maximize vegetable intake. Healthy fats are encouraged, along with moderate protein.

7. During maintenance, work up to a 16:8 approach: a sixteen-hour overnight fast and an eight-hour eating window. For instance, eat at 10 a.m., finish by 6 p.m., and eat no food between 6 p.m. that day and 10 a.m. the next day.

8. You can pick your own feeding window as long as it allows for a sixteen-hour overnight fast. Most of my patients find it easiest to track this with an app. Working women or those who socialize a lot at dinner often prefer a later eating window, say, noon to 8 p.m. (Note that some women need to stick to 14:10 for one week before extending to 16:8 if sixteen hours feels stressful or too long at first. You can ease into it.)

9. Time the taking of your early morning and bedtime probiotics to help to boost the anti-obesogenic bacteria and reduce the obesogenic bacteria (in, for example, the *Lactobacillus* family).

10. Continue circadian-based intermittent fasting past the four-week Gottfried Protocol if you've got more than 15 pounds to lose.

## Daily Checklist for the Gottfried Protocol

- Bowel movement.
- Weight recorded.
- Blood ketones and glucose tested to determine GKI.
- Circadian-based intermittent fasting.
- Sweating (daily body movement — fasted workouts are best — and an Epsom salt bath or a sauna five days per week).
- Hydration with added no-sugar electrolytes to support kidney function, reduce risk of kidney stones, and prevent "keto flu."
- Continual detoxification through eating vegetables, avoiding toxins, and encouraging balanced liver function.

# Q&A WITH DR. SARA

**Q:** *I have (fill in the blank with a medical condition). Can I do the Gottfried Protocol?*

**A:** Unfortunately, it is not possible to cover in this book every possible medical condition and whether it contraindicates ketosis. Also, I cannot give specific medical advice outside an established patient-physician relationship. Instead, I encourage you to consult with a member of your health-care team, such as your primary care physician. The contraindications to the ketogenic diet that I discuss in Chapter 4, both in the text and the Notes, are a start. But to find out what will work specifically for you, it's best to get advice from medical professionals who know you.

## THE TOP SEVEN THINGS
## THAT GO SIDEWAYS ON
## THE GOTTFRIED PROTOCOL

Because I've been using this program with patients, I've encountered many common problems that can derail success. Here's what to look out for and how to respond:

1. **You eat too many calories.** When I first tried keto, I had difficulty achieving my macros, so I starting drinking my coffee with butter and MCT oil. I was consuming too much fat and eating beyond my metabolic ceiling. You may overeat because you are leptin resistant and you do not feel full, even in ketosis. (You can check for this by measuring your leptin level in the blood. If above 8 ng/dL, leptin resistance may be driving you to overeat.) The solution is to eat foods that are lower in calorie density. Greens (such as salads) have 100 calories per pound. Vegetables, 200 calories per pound. Meat has 800 calories, bread 1,500, and chocolate 2,500 calories per pound. Calorie-

dense foods activate the reward system.[31] Eat more greens and vegetables, and less meat.

2. **You keep drinking alcohol.** Do you want to burn fat, improve your sleep, and clear your brain, or do you want to drink your glass of wine? I'll wait here while that reality check sinks in. In my experience, alcohol will kick you out of ketosis. And it certainly disrupts most of your hormones. Take 1–2 teaspoons of MCT in the afternoon to avoid that first glass of wine. Based on anecdotal reports, it seems to raise healthy short-chain fatty acids in the body, which may make you feel more satisfied when you prepare for dinner.[32]

3. **You have a slow metabolism.** We know that women with a higher BMI and slower metabolic rate (the rate at which you burn calories at rest) take longer to lose weight and may be more likely to experience plateaus. Improving hormonal balance may take longer, but it may help with boosting metabolic rate. You may want to seek professional help to measure your resting metabolic rate and test hormones.

4. **You experience constipation.** This is a common side effect of ketosis. I've seen patients retain or gain 2 to 5 pounds due to constipation, even when they are having a partial bowel movement each morning. The problem may be incomplete bowel evacuation. Try the techniques listed on page 146 if this happens to you.

5. **You have trouble getting into ketosis.** Or perhaps you get into ketosis but come back out of it. There can be several reasons for this, including eating too much protein. The amount of protein you ate ten or twenty years ago may no longer be the right amount for you. If, in my fifties, I ate the same level of protein that I did when I was in my thirties, I would have high blood sugar now. Other common foods that may spike your blood sugar and lower your level of ketosis are dairy products, alternative sweeteners, alcohol, and packaged foods. (Recently, I used a tooth whitener from my dentist, which popped me out of ketosis and caused my fasting glucose to rise to the 110

mg/dL range, which is where I used to be back when I had prediabetes.) For optimal therapeutic benefits, I'd like for you to get in and stay in ketosis for four weeks. When in doubt, test. The best way to know if a food is suppressing ketosis is to test your ketones and glucose before and after eating the food. I like to test before eating it and again one hour after, and once more two hours later. See more detail in the next chapter, where we further discuss how to identify your trigger foods and determine your personal carb limit.

6. **You have a high level of carb intolerance.** You may need to drop total carbs further, down to 5 percent of total calories per day. True, I've given you all the reasons why this may not be good for your hormones, but the kingpin hormone is insulin, and we need to get that hormone straightened out first.

7. **You come down with a case of the "f*ck its."** Oh, I've been there. Maybe you're constantly hungry because steady ketosis hasn't yet kicked in (probably due to item 5 or 6 in this list). Maybe your metabolism is on the slow side, so weight loss is more gradual than you want. Maybe you're sick of diet culture or berating yourself over eating too much. The goal here isn't to make you unhealthfully thin; instead, the objective is to swap your badly behaved hormones for hormones that optimize your health and help you accomplish your long-term vision for yourself. For me, that means a healthy BMI, with good muscle tone and all the clothes in the closet fitting well. Getting dressed is simple. Food is neutral. I can go four to six hours between meals, with steady blood sugar and energy. I've waited most of my life for this level of freedom and security, and I want that for you too.

## Nine Plateau Busters

If your weight seems stuck going up and down within a 2- to 3-pound range and won't drop after five to seven days, consider trying one of these:

1. Resistance training. Aim for two-thirds weight training and one-third cardio. Lift heavy weights. Building muscle will raise your resting metabolic rate. Bonus: exercise when you first wake up, before your eating window opens.
2. Using a food scale. Weighing your food will keep you honest and on track.
3. Mitochondrial support. I recommend taking L-carnitine first thing in the morning to help transport triglycerides to your mitochondria, where fat is burned.
4. Cryotherapy. This is exposure to cold air or water. I go to a local cryotherapy center. Or you could take an ice bath (a cold bath with ice) for 20 minutes twice per week. Some people prefer cold showers.
5. Troubleshooting net carbs. If you're not losing weight, drop your net carbs below 20 grams per day to combat carb intolerance or insulin resistance. Consider getting a blood test to look at fasting insulin, glucose, and hemoglobin A1C. The good news is that once you use this food plan to reverse your carb intolerance, you will be able to eat more carbs without gaining weight.
6. Restricting calories. Try doing this temporarily, for one to two days.
7. Extending fasting. Go for 18:6 or even 20:4.
8. Adding insulin sensitizers. These supplements may improve the function of insulin and improve fat loss. (See page 159 for details about keto-supportive supplements.)
9. Adding growth-hormone-boosting peptides. They require a prescription and a responsible prescriber, but they may help when nothing else is working.

What if you can't get into ketosis? Here are good strategies to kick your body into ketosis if you're not getting there:

- Try cryotherapy (see Plateau Busters).
- Add fat, like extra-virgin olive oil.
- Restrict calories, or fast for fourteen to sixteen hours to flip the metabolic switch to the fat-burning mode.
- Incorporate MCT oil (40 grams per day can induce ketosis).
- Try additional blood sugar support (see the box below for details about keto-supportive supplements).

What if you're constipated? Regular bowel movements are key to your success. Here are some great tricks to help you avoid or do away with constipation, a common issue for women on keto plans:

- Hydrate adequately.
- Eat high-fiber vegetables plus 25 grams of lettuce daily (any type of lettuce; see Recipes for ideas).
- Consume one quarter of an avocado.
- Eat ground flaxseed.
- Take MCT oil.
- Add a magnesium supplement.

## Keto-Supportive Supplements

Evidence from scientific studies shows that these supplements help resolve inflammation. Consider them in addition to the supplements I mentioned previously to support the liver.

- **Alpha-lipoic acid** is a fatty acid made by your body, and I recommend it in supplement form to encourage weight loss and improve insulin sensitivity; solid evidence points to its effectiveness in preventing cell damage in the body.[33] I prescribe this supplement for prediabetes, diabetes, aging skin, lipid problems, cataracts, glaucoma, and other health issues. It enhances insulin sensitivity, lowers glucose, and reduces advanced glycation end products (AGEs, harmful substances formed when protein or fat combine with sugar in the body).[34] It can help you with age-related loss in glutathione, the master antioxidant. Alpha-lipoic acid improves mitochondria. (See Resources; there are two forms, or isomers, which have different properties, and I recommend R-lipoic acid because it is more biologically active than S-lipoic acid. Alpha-lipoic acid supplements tend to include the "R" and "S" forms in a 50:50 ratio.) A dose of R-lipoic acid is 100 to 200 milligrams per day, with 2–4 milligrams of biotin per day as well, to prevent the biotin depletion that can occur with long-term use of lipoic acid.

- **Balanced omegas** — you need to be well oiled to resolve inflammation.[35] I recommend taking a blend of different omegas, including alpha linoleic acid, eicosapentaenoic acid (EPA), docosahexaenoic acid (DHA), which are omega-3s, and gamma linoleic acid, a healthy omega-6. Therapy with just one of these may create an imbalance in your fatty acid pathway. For my patients, I track the ratio of omega-3 to omega-6 because higher ratios are associated with lower risk of disease (or conversely, we seek lower ratios if looking at the ratio of omega-6 to omega-3), including breast cancer.[36] See Resources for further information.

- **Berberine** has been shown to lower blood sugar and inflammation, and to modestly reduce weight.[37] Dose: 500 milligrams, three times per day.

- **Specialized proresolving mediators (SPMs)** are a recent discovery that may help with the chronic inflammation of insulin resistance and obesity, though randomized trials have not been performed.[38] See Resources for dosing details.

- **Spirulina** is a type of blue-green algae that I add to my shakes, as you will see in the Recipe section. A dose of 500 milligrams twice per day (or the approximate equivalent in your daily shake) is associated with lower weight and appetite. Spirulina is anti-inflammatory and detoxifying.

# Common Hormone Imbalances: PCOS and Breast Cancer

The most common hormone imbalance that I see in my medical practice is polycystic ovary syndrome (PCOS), affecting 20 to 30 percent of my patients. Women with PCOS are the most resistant to weight loss because they are battling multiple hormone problems at once: insulin block, leptin resistance, low adiponectin (a hormone derived from fat that protects against insulin resistance, diabetes, and atherosclerosis), high testosterone and DHEA, high cortisol, high aromatase, and, as a result, dysestrogenism (known colloquially as "estrogen dominance"). They have signs of unresolved inflammation, like belly fat, and blood tests showing high cRP, interleukin-6, and TNF-alpha, which raise aromatase and put weight loss even further out of reach.

Back in 2013, I recommended a low-carb diet full of whole foods and polyphenols to address PCOS, as that was the most well proven approach at the time, and this was further validated since the publication of my book *The Hormone Cure*.[39] Fortunately, we now have more data to support a hormone-balancing ketogenic diet for women struggling with PCOS, with studies showing weight loss and improved hormones, from insulin to testosterone.[40]

What about breast cancer, the dreaded disease that affects one in eight women within the course of a lifetime? PCOS has many risk factors that overlap with those of breast cancer, and the hormonal pattern in PCOS may be implicated in the development of breast cancer: specifically, wayward insulin.[41] (Studies that try to correlate PCOS with breast cancer are mixed — some positive[42] and some negative[43] — though the negative studies failed to make appropriate statistical adjustments.) Meta-analyses show a definitive link between PCOS and endometrial cancer, another hormonally mediated type of cancer.[44] The takeaway is that the hormone-balancing keto reset is a well-documented way to address metabolic dysfunction, the root cause of both PCOS and breast cancer.

# *Highlights*

► In this chapter, you learned to layer in deeper detoxification and periods of metabolic rest by fasting each night for fourteen to sixteen hours.

► Together we can troubleshoot the most common problems that arise on a hormone-balancing ketogenic diet to maintain the four-week pulse and keep you burning fat and losing weight.

► You gained weight gradually, and you will lose weight gradually. Go slowly. Keep the long view. Aim for long-term weight loss and maintenance. You'll have to do this only once if you do it right.

► You don't have to be perfect — stress resulting from perfectionism raises cortisol and insulin, and can block weight loss — but you can't quit. Not now, not before you receive all the demonstrated benefits of a well-formulated ketogenic diet that balances your hormones and makes you feel more alive.

► Reread Chapter 5 and this chapter for the support you need. Go to my Instagram (Instagram.com/saragottfriedmd) to ask questions and be part of the community of Gottfried Protocol warriors.

# 7

## TRANSITION

You did it! You spent four weeks reorganizing, recovering, and restoring your hormones to create metabolic youth. You followed the rules and made it to Day 29. I've been there myself, and I know that road can be challenging. Your hormone levels, hormone receptors, and transportation of hormones in your body are all improved, and as a result you've lost weight and feel like yourself again. It's a process of deconstructing the old version of your body and reconstituting it in a superior way. Congratulations!

**Preparation**
20–25 grams of net carbs and detoxification. Keep a ketogenic ratio of 2:1. Get your bowels moving so you can mobilize fat!

**Implementation**
20–25 grams net carbs per day, and add intermittent fasting (14/10 to 16/8). Continue a ketogenic ratio of 2:1.

**Transition**
Start to add net carbs slowly, 5 grams at a time, and heading toward a ketogenic ratio of 1:1 for the long term, or until you repeat the diet.

The Gottfried Protocol Timeline

I've seen over the years in my practice that getting your hormones back in balance is one of the best actions you can take to promote long-term health and to feel incredible. Still, most people don't realize that making a significant lifestyle change, even for a pulse of four weeks, presents a major psychosocial challenge. Your partner probably complained or gave you an eye roll. Maybe you're weary of making multiple meals for others at home and along with yours. You probably want to skip meal prep on Sunday. By this stage of the program, I hope you realize the pounds lost don't matter as much as your mindset — your self-directed attitude and thoughts. Most important, how do you feel? On Day 29, I expect that you feel triumphant, regardless of whether your progress with weight loss was big or small. I agree: it was the tiny steps you took each day that added up over four weeks to major transformation.

The intention of the Gottfried Protocol is to change the conversation between your food and hormones. By Day 29, you've started a new conversation between your hormones and fat to make you leaner and healthier. You are creating metabolic flexibility, the ability of your body to efficiently switch between using carbs and fats as fuel, based on your need and available nutrients. The whole point is to not be trapped in the metabolically inflexible state of burning carbs 24/7. Maybe your brain fog cleared up, your night sweats and hot flashes are ebbing, or your PCOS symptoms are improving. You're now burning more fat and feeling hopeful and encouraged about weight loss.

So, what's next?

During Transition, you will be burning both fat and carbs to meet your body's energy demand, and we will define the upper and lower limit of the amount of carbs that works best for you, for continued fat burning. Transition takes about a week or two, and it will provide a lifetime of benefits.

## MEET LOTUS, AGE FIFTY-ONE

Lotus is a busy physician who went on the Gottfried Protocol to deal with her growing waistline, slowing metabolism, and worsening cholesterol levels. Before we met, her hormones had felt like a hot mess for many months. Previously, she suffered from endometriosis and underwent a hysterectomy and ovary removal in 2019. She had all the symptoms of perimenopause: weight gain, hot flashes, night sweats, brain fog, and mood swings. Her thyroid function was slow; she had prediabetes. At a height of 5 feet, 4 inches, and a weight of 163 pounds, she had an overweight body mass index of 28. Combined with a low metabolic rate (a calculated basal metabolic rate of 1,406 calories/day), this meant slower progress with the Gottfried Protocol, but Lotus prevailed. She had tried a ketogenic diet before, but it didn't work — she felt she never had effective guidance or the right mindset. After I explained the Protocol and walked her through the guidelines I share in this book, she felt ready.

Three weeks later, Lotus was making great progress. All of her perimenopausal symptoms were gone, a result I see frequently because those symptoms are driven by hormones — not just estrogen and progesterone but insulin too.[1]

After four weeks, Lotus was down to 154 pounds (and had a lower BMI of 26) and felt a renewed sense of grace, like she had a new lease on life. She kept to her 2:1 ketogenic ratio with mostly vegetarian Indian food. (I include several of her recipes in Chapter 9.) When she checked her labs before and after the Gottfried Protocol, her leptin and testosterone were normal, her blood sugar was improved, her total cholesterol had dropped, and her good cholesterol was the best it had been in twelve years. Progress!

We still need to work on her fitness, muscle mass, and growth hormone to build on her amazing gains. Our new goal became to get her BMI to less than 24.9 and to increase growth hormone with weight training. Meanwhile, at the time of this writing, she has lost 39 pounds, her weight is 124 pounds, she has a BMI of 21.3, and her GKI is consistently 2–3. Now our goal is maintenance, with added carbs and more exercise. She has her energy back and has found a new balance and joy.

## HANDLE YOUR
## TRANSITION WITH CARE

Like Lotus, you'll take on the final task in the Gottfried Protocol, which is to protect your new hormones by slowly transitioning to a more balanced food plan. As I mentioned in the introduction, the Gottfried Protocol is a therapeutic pulse to right your hormones, not a long-term diet. We just don't have enough data related to women to recommend it for an extended period.

I know you are eager to be done, but I urge you to move through this final stage with great patience and grace. In this chapter, I will teach you how to gradually increase your carbohydrates while staying on the edge of ketosis. The Gottfried Protocol is a food plan meant to be followed for four weeks, and a maximum of six months continuously, before easing into a more evidence-based, balanced, and anti-inflammatory food plan, such as the Mediterranean diet. (I will cover this transition in this chapter.)

If you finish your four weeks of the Gottfried Protocol and then on Day 29 splurge on 200 grams of carbs, you will lose the sacred opportunity to learn the upper and lower limit of the carb threshold that works for you. Reintroduce additional carbs slowly, and be patient. If you return to all the old carbs you used to eat, you will both lose this opportunity and gain back the weight you lost.

The Transition phase of adding back carbohydrates may take you nine days, or it may take you longer. Everyone is unique. Don't skimp on it. Don't race through it with a plate of nachos and multiple rounds of margaritas. Take the time you need to collect data on yourself and then integrate this information. I will take you by the hand and show you how to do it methodically, based on my latest experience with transitioning off a ketogenic food plan over the past several years. The goal is to be like Lotus, who has transitioned to a mostly vegetarian and balanced diet with more carbs and less fat, yet continues to stay in mild ketosis and lose weight. Despite many health challenges, like a slow metabolic rate and a BMI in the overweight range, Lotus is down 39 pounds from when she started. She feels hopeful for the first time in years, which empowers her to keep working for better health.

## RULES OF ENGAGEMENT FOR TRANSITION

Our main goal of Transition is to define your carb limit so that you can determine an upper limit on the carbohydrates you can eat each day and not gain weight. In the process, you will learn about digestion, absorption, focus, mood, energy, performance, sleep, self-care, and health versus disease. We all have our own carb threshold for weight loss. The healthier you get, the higher the number. These rules of engagement will help you define your personal carb limit to enable you to maintain healthy hormones and continue to lose weight.

- **Define your carb limit.** This will be the number of daily net carbs under which you will continue to lose weight and over which you may begin to gain weight.
- **Continue measuring ketones.** Stay in mild ketosis either with the food that you eat, or with circadian fasting, or ideally, with both. Keep up the detoxification: this has been shown to improve metabolic flexibility by relying less on glucose and more on ketones. Over the long term, mild ketosis is one of the best ways to improve health span, the period of time you are free of disease and feeling your healthiest.[2]
- **Transfer to an anti-inflammatory diet**. I recommend a carb-adjusted version of the evidence-based Mediterranean diet (more details later in this chapter). You will be able to manage your weight successfully because you'll know your personal carb limit, and if you need to continue to lose weight, you'll repeat the four-week pulse of the Gottfried Protocol after you finish Transition. Armed with your carb limit, you can continue to lose weight by staying below it.

- **If you fall out of ketosis, get back in as soon as possible.** If you are still craving more carbs or processed food, it can take longer than twenty-eight days to adapt to ketosis and rid yourself of cravings. Just because you're in ketosis doesn't mean all cravings disappear. For some of my patients, it takes a few days, but for others, it can take months. Of course, you are not defined by the number on the bathroom scale or the size of your dress. You are defined by your daily choices, particularly what you do when faced with a challenge. Think of indulging a craving as a challenge, nothing more, nothing less. I like to have a plan for when I fall off the wagon — and I'll share my best strategies with you later in this chapter.

- **Keep your motivation in mind.** Remember why you embarked on the Gottfried Protocol: to change your relationship to carbs and to fix your hormones. We all know the allure of carbs. One bite may feel soothing, but the truth is, most forms of carbohydrate — whether it's popcorn, starchy foods (rice, potatoes, root vegetables), fructose (fruit sugar), lactose (milk sugar), or sugar itself (and its cousins: honey, maple syrup, and even some sugar substitutes) — turn into glucose in the gut. Excess carbs are the root cause of hormone imbalance for many people. Unfortunately, the more you eat, the more you want. Stand firm as you test your carb limits, and follow the plan I describe in this chapter. Keep in mind that when you overeat carbs, you convert your body back into a fat-storing machine. Avoid the hormonal mess that leads to diabetes and metabolic syndrome by carefully titrating your own personal carb limit.

## DEFINE YOUR CARB LIMIT

The Gottfried Protocol starts you at a carb limit of 20 to 25 net carbs per day. For the first three days of Transition, increase your net carbs by 5 grams. It may take up to three days to notice a change in your weight or other measures (listed below). If your weight stays the same or decreases, after three days add another 5 grams, and track how your body responds over the next three days.

For example, if you were eating 20 grams of net carbs per day for the four weeks of the Gottfried Protocol, then for Days 29–31, eat 25 grams of net carbs. If you stay in ketosis and your weight stays stable or continues to decrease, then on Days 32–35, eat 30 grams of net carbs. On Days 36–39, eat 35 grams of net carbs. Track your weight, blood sugar, and ketones each day. When your weight increases, you've reached your personal carb limit.

Your blood ketones will probably decrease as you reach your carb limit. When you fall out of ketosis (blood ketones less than 0.5 mmol/L) and your weight loss stops, you have reached your personal carb limit. Dial your daily carb limit to less than this threshold.

What carbs should you add first? I recommend adding starchier vegetables first, then low-sugar fruits such as berries, along with legumes and hummus. Be very careful with potatoes, grains, and dairy until your personal carb limit is well defined.

## What Determines Your Personal Carb Limit?

- Current weight.
- Gender.
- Health and lifestyle.
- Genetics and epigenetics (how the genes talk to your cells).
- Glucose and ketones.
- Hormones like insulin, cortisol, growth hormone, leptin.
- Age.
- Metabolic flexibility.
- Foods you eat — before and during the Gottfried Protocol.
- Stress level.
- Gut function.
- Level of physical activity.
- Medications.

## Signs That You've Exceeded
## Your Personal Carb Limit

- **Increase in weight.** Normally weight can fluctuate by about 1 pound per day when hormones are stable. If you are having a daily bowel movement and your weight increases by 2 pounds or more over the next seventy-two hours, you've crossed your current carb limit.
- **Rise in glucose (fasting glucose greater than 85 mg/dL) and decline in ketones (less than 0.5 mmol/L).** This represents a fasting glucose-ketone index greater than 10.
- **Fatigue.** When you go past your carb limit, you may feel exhausted, like you need a nap. Depending on when you consume the extra carbs, fatigue could occur in the morning, afternoon, or evening, or all day long. Usually the fatigue occurs after the meal with excess carbs.
- **Brain fog.** Overconsumption of carbs may cause difficulty with focus or concentration. This is one of the most common symptoms of insulin resistance.
- **Mood swings.** Excess carbs can make you feel depressed or tired.
- **Bloating.** Eating over your personal carb limit may cause intestinal gas.

## How Much Is 5 Net Carbs?

Okay, now you know the plan — here's what those 5 net carbs look like on your plate:

- 2 ounces of butternut squash. I cut fresh squash into cubes and store them in the freezer so I can steam small amounts at a time.
- ½ of a sweet potato (1.75 ounces), which has about 8 net carbs; aim for 1 ounce only.
- ¼ cup of blueberries, which contains about 4 to 5 net carbs.
- ¼ cup of black beans, which contains 5.8 net carbs, so eat a little less (approximately 1 ounce).

- 1 ounce cashews (28 grams), or about 18, which contain 7.7 grams of net carbs. I'll do the math for you: eat 11 cashews to get 5 net carbs.
- 1 piece of keto bread (my favorite has 4 net carbs; see Resources).

## CHECK FOR FOOD INTOLERANCES

Consider testing certain foods to see if you are intolerant to them by measuring whether they block your ketone levels. Many foods trigger ketone dips or glucose spikes for some people but not for others. These are common culprits:

- Dairy products.
- Grains.
- Gluten.
- Egg.
- Alcohol.
- Artificial sweeteners.
- Legumes.
- Almond or coconut flour.
- Rice.
- Prepackaged foods.

One of the best ways to tell if you're reacting to a specific food is to measure your ketones and glucose before and after you eat it. It's a three-test process (described in the next section), but it's worth the extra effort because once you know which food is getting in your way, you can eliminate it from your diet. Why does this matter? Because food intolerances can lead to weight-loss resistance and autoimmune disease. The most frequent food intolerances found in a recent study of a hundred people with autoimmune conditions were casein, cow's milk, wheat, gliadin (a type of protein in gluten), egg whites, and rice.[3]

I know what you're thinking: what about your bones? Dairy may not do your body good, despite the marketing messages from the

Dairy Council. A new study found that dairy products do not prevent age-related bone loss or fractures in women over age forty.[4] Great sources of calcium include many of the Gottfried Protocol foods, like cruciferous vegetables (collard greens, broccoli, and kale), eggs, greens (such as spinach), and sesame seeds. Also, I tell my patients to maintain healthy levels of vitamin D (serum levels of 50–90 ng/mL) to ensure bone strength and to let this vitamin handle the approximately 399 jobs it does for us, such as immune system modulation.

A note about alcohol: When you've been off alcohol for three or more weeks, your liver is clean and fresh. Drinking will hit you harder than before. If you choose to reintroduce alcohol, start with half a serving, such as about 2.5 ounces of wine.

## CONTINUE MEASURING KETONES

As you become more keto-adapted, you will continue to improve your metabolic flexibility and become more efficient at burning both carbs and fat. In Transition, keep tracking your macronutrients (fat, protein, total carbs, net carbs), daily weight, weekly waist circumference, ketones, and potentially your glucose-ketone index (GKI).

We can use GKI to track your body's response to an increase in carb intake. We want your ketones to continue to be 0.5 to 3.0 millimolar per liter (mmol/L). A blood ketone level that is less than 0.5 mmol/L means the body is not in ketosis.

During Transition, I measure my ketones and glucose first thing in the morning after weighing myself, and again after eating a test food of extra net carbs. Like me, you can check postprandial GKI one and two hours after you eat to test for food intolerances (read on for more details on this).

As we discussed, GKI is one of the best indicators of your metabolic state. Continue to aim for a GKI of 1–3 to address obesity, insulin resistance (block), and weight loss. A GKI of 3–6 is still helpful for repairing insulin block, and a GKI of 6–9 still has weight-loss benefits.

# MEASURING FOR FOOD INTOLERANCES

To tell if you're reacting to a specific food as a food intolerance or sensitivity, perform the following three-step process:

1. Measure your fasting (or preprandial, "before meal") glucose and ketones; this should be done at least three hours after your last meal. Then determine your GKI. This is your baseline.
2. Eat or drink the food in question. It's best if you eat only this food, such as a serving of yogurt, cheese, or beans.
3. Measure your glucose and ketones again 60 minutes and then 120 minutes later. Calculate the GKI.

How to interpret the results: Avoid foods that cause your blood glucose to rise more than 30 mg/dL from baseline to the 60-minute result or prevent it from returning to baseline after two hours. Ideally your glucose should be between 90 and 115 mg/dL. Limit or avoid foods that cause a drop in ketones of 0.5–1.0 mmol/L, or less than 0.5 mmol/L, or a GKI greater than 10, or some combination of these results.

# BENEFITS OF THE MEDITERRANEAN DIET

The Mediterranean diet is an ancient way of eating that evolved in the region of the Mediterranean Sea, particularly Italy and Greece, which boast the healthiest and longest-lived populations in the world. As you transition from the four-week Gottfried Protocol to a Mediterranean diet, you will have many more food options, and you can modulate the amount of carbs you consume each day (since you know your personal carb limit) by eating just below your limit.

These are the foods featured in the Mediterranean diet:

- Plant-based whole foods (nuts, seeds, vegetables, fruits, legumes, grains).

- Moderate consumption of fish, seafood, and dairy.
- Limited red meat and other meat products.
- Olive oil as the main source of fat and cooking oil.
- Low-to-moderate consumption of alcohol, mostly red wine (as my patients are quick to point out).

Indigenous edible plants and herbs from the region include olives, borage, chard, capers, lupines, asparagus, watercress, mallow, thistle, grapes, beets, tigernut, parsley, cumin, coriander, fennel, oregano, rosemary, sage, lemon balm, savory, fenugreek, bay leaf, saffron, and mushrooms. Other plants originated in Asia (rice, fruits like apples, raspberries, plum, quince), Africa (artichoke, millet, okra, melons), and the Americas (corn, peanuts, tomatoes, peppers, eggplant).[5]

Multiple randomized trials have shown the health benefits of a Mediterranean diet for risk reduction of cardiovascular disease,[6] metabolic syndrome,[7] type 2 diabetes,[8] obesity,[9] cancer[10] (including breast cancer),[11] cognitive decline,[12] and other neurodegenerative disease like Alzheimer's[13] and multiple sclerosis.[14] Specifically, for the best blood sugar control in diabetes, the Mediterranean diet and the low-carb diet are equally effective at reducing glycated hemoglobin (known as a blood test called hemoglobin A1C) and weight, together with providing the greatest benefit in high-density lipoprotein (the "good" cholesterol).[15]

Personally, I gain weight on a classic Mediterranean diet because I have a low personal carb limit. If that's the case for you, focus during Transition on a low-carb Mediterranean diet, limiting grains and fruit and loading up on vegetables, nuts, seeds, fish, and seafood.

## Alcohol: My Opinion

My opinion on alcohol is not popular. But the truth is, the very thing that we hope to get from alcohol — relaxation, relief from the stress of a busy day — is getting robbed from us. Most patients I guide through the Gottfried Protocol are eager to get back on booze. Most patients I talk to about transitioning to the Mediterranean diet interrupt me to sing the praises of red wine. I urge caution because that eagerness may signal a sticky relationship to alcohol, which may slow down or even halt your progress with hormone balancing and ketosis.

What does alcohol do to the body? Two glasses of Chardonnay contain more than 6 grams of carbs, and after being on the wagon for four weeks, your liver is clearer and alcohol can take it down, making you buzzed faster. Alcohol raises cortisol, which may then disrupt your sleep. This has a knock-on effect on insulin. We know that one night of bad sleep makes you more insulin resistant the next day. Higher cortisol may disrupt the regular insulin signal. If you are chronically disrupting it by consuming a moderate amount of alcohol, that will lead to more insulin resistance. Add to that high stress, not getting enough exercise to make your muscles hungry for glucose, and you start to get a compounded problem with insulin.

Simply put, alcohol can harm your hormones.[16] Alcohol is a neurotoxin. After ages thirty-five to forty, the blood-brain barrier (BBB) gets thinner, so alcohol hits harder and hangovers linger longer. Additionally, alcohol can alter the BBB by changing the normal function of your tight junctions. A leaky blood-brain barrier is linked to multiple problems, such as memory issues, multiple sclerosis, stroke, and Alzheimer's disease. Plus, alcohol is a carcinogen that increases a woman's risk of breast cancer, even at the modest dose of three servings per week.

Alcohol wreaks havoc on the liver, your primary detox organ. Alcohol is the toxin that goes to the front of the line in liver metabolism. It's like a triage system. Ridding alcohol from your system is your liver's top priority. That means that all the other toxins we are exposed to that we can't avoid — such as air pollutants and pesticides — get pushed to the back of the detox line when alcohol is around.

Half of US adults drink alcohol, and 10 percent have alcohol use disorder (AUD). Women get buzzed and drunk faster than men, even when adjusted for body weight, because we have more fat and less water, and there are other variations based on the menstrual cycle. Historically, alcohol misuse and AUD have been more common in men than women. However, recent data from the past ten years show we are catching up. The alcohol industry specifically targets women in their marketing campaigns and wants to normalize alcohol consumption, so that you feel it is a core part of feeling good and connected to others.

Binge eating is associated with AUD,[17] so if you want to correct your hormones and feel your best, limit or eliminate the alcohol. I encourage you to assess your relationship with alcohol honestly and reconsider whether it is good for your health, particularly after age thirty-five. Don't fall for the lie that Big Alcohol is telling you and that perhaps your friends have internalized.

## KEEP DETOXING

By Day 29, you will have cleared out many toxic fats by following the Gottfried Protocol. Consuming healthy fats like olive oil, avocado oil, nuts, and seeds — along with fiber — will help you flush out the liver and gallbladder and rid toxic fats (from trans fats, fried foods, and excessive saturated fat) from your body. The job of the gallbladder is to break down fats after a meal. Eating healthy fat will trigger the hormone cholecystokinin to nudge the gallbladder to collect bile and release it into the intestines to improve digestion of fat. If you have had your gallbladder removed or have gallbladder issues, you may find that you digest MCT oil best because it is broken down more easily.

Some of my patients continue to have occasional constipation, and I repeat the same recommendations:

- Aim to evacuate fully your bowels a minimum of once (or twice) per day.
- Drink plenty of water, and add no-sugar electrolytes.
- Eat high-fiber vegetables, including lettuces and cruciferous vegetables.
- Add ground flaxseed and/or MCT oil to each meal.
- Take your magnesium — most of us are low, so I try to get my Gottfried Protocol participants up to 800 milligrams per day.
- Continue exercising and sweating — they will help you maintain your fat loss.

## CONTINUE CIRCADIAN-BASED INTERMITTENT FASTING

You've now had firsthand experience in how effective intermittent fasting is, and, if you're like most of my patients, you probably find that it's a relatively easy lifestyle shift to make. That should be motivation enough to continue intermittent fasting through Transition and beyond. Your commitment will be met with improved insulin, growth hormone and other hormones, fat loss, and increased energy, vitality, and focus.

Throughout Transition, continue with the sixteen-hour overnight fast for about two to five days per week. Some of our Gottfried Protocol participants do it every night to keep their blood sugar, insulin, and ketosis in the optimal range. Hormones are released on a circadian rhythm, and you can keep yours releasing correctly by getting 10 minutes of morning light before 10 a.m., which helps raise melatonin at night and strengthens your hormonal rhythm. I do this with

## Decision Tree for Transition

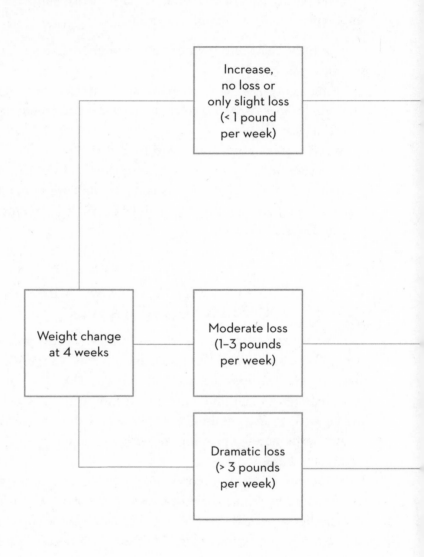

Honesty check:
are you cheating?

**Yes** → Connect to values and find that core reason that you really want to lose weight and try again.

Are you exercising enough? Increase activity levels with yoga, pilates, or walking.

**No** → Increase vegetable consumption while decreasing fat consumption to reduce total calories without hunger.

Is your thyroid functioning properly? Ask your doctor to test for free T4, anti-TPO antibodies, and TSH.

→ Reduce carb consumption to crescendo levels.

Are your stress levels high and sleep poor? Increase exercise levels, develop a relaxing pre-sleep routine, and eat dinner earlier.

→ Nutrition: can you increase nutrient quality in your food choices — like replacing processed meats with simple high-quality meat?

Great! Continue with Gottfried Protocol.

**No** → Increase carb consumption by 5g/day with foods like sweet potatoes, squash, avocado, and fruit.

→ Reduce activity/exercise levels if high.

Do you feel healthy, energetic, and inspired?

**Yes** → Continue Gottfried Protocol, but monitor energy and adjust if energy declines.

a dog walk most mornings. Continue circadian-based intermittent fasting past the four-week Gottfried Protocol if you've got more than 15 pounds to lose.

## WHAT TO DO AFTER FALLING OFF THE WAGON

Look, it happens. Maybe it was a holiday splurge or a birthday celebration. At some point, you may find that you've overindulged in foods that take you out of ketosis and make you gain weight. When that happens, get back on the path as soon as possible. Return to your personal carb limit and aim below it. I advise my patients to plan their recovery meals in advance — Gottfried Protocol–compliant meals that will help you regain a sense of balance. To avoid further temptation and get back on track, make a contract with yourself. Start implementing it the day after your overindulgence. Here is a simple outline you can use:

Personal carb limit _____

Eating window _____

Breakfast _____

Lunch _____

Dinner _____

Exercise goal _____

Weight the next day _____

## LAST THOUGHTS ON TRANSITION

As a final sendoff, remember to feed and nurture yourself. Have you taken my advice to find your favorite ways to hit the pause button? Found an app that supports you? Sometimes I need a daily reminder to reconsent to this process. I feel too busy to slow down, but we need to slow down in order for healing to occur. All healing takes place in the parasympathetic nervous system, where relaxation, deep belly breathing, and chilling out are the focus.

I believe the body is on loan from a Higher Power, so don't you want to take every measure to care for it? I know I do, and that's what I hope for my patients and tribe. That includes metabolic flexibility — your capacity to adapt to burning carbs or fat based on fuel availability.

Continue aiming for a BMI of 18.5 to 24.9 kg/m², but remember to break it down into modules. We discussed Lara's modules for weight loss in the last chapter; her initial goal or module was to lose 5 pounds of mostly fat in order to get her BMI to less than 24.9 kg/m².

For Lotus, the first module was the same as Lara's: to lose 5 pounds of mostly fat. The second module was to complete four weeks of the Gottfried Protocol, in which she lost a cumulative total of 12.5 pounds. The third module was to get her BMI under 24.9 during Transition while slowly switching to a lower-carbohydrate Mediterranean diet. In Transition, Lotus began to back off from the ketogenic ratio of 2:1 so we could see how her body (and weight) would respond to incrementally higher carb levels; this occasionally put her into a ketogenic ratio of 1:1. She even enjoyed a small piece of chocolate cake at her daughter's birthday celebration, but she got right back on plan with her next meal — and has lost a total of 33 pounds. A reasonable goal is to be like Lotus and continue to lose 3 to 5 pounds of mostly fat per month after you complete the Gottfried Protocol.

What's it worth to have the healthiest version of your body? I place the highest value on it, a higher value than the slight awkwardness of declining noncompliant food or alcohol when I'm visiting with friends, or the temptation when my daughter orders pizza. You won't feel your best if you are chronically inflamed, overwhelmed, depleted, or stressed. Take the time to perform Transition carefully and methodically in order to reach a level of health and vigor that you may not have known was possible for you.

# *Highlights*

▶ In this chapter, we discussed reintroducing small doses of carbohydrates in order to define your personal carb limit. Take it step by step, or 5 grams of net carbs at a time, to determine your threshold for weight loss going forward.

▶ You may also choose to reintroduce alcohol and see how you respond to it, but be cautious and lower your dose — your liver pathways are now clear and alcohol will hit harder.

▶ Watch out for foods that spike your blood sugar or take you out of ketosis by tracking your glucose-ketone index. When you identify problem foods and eliminate them, you set yourself up for long-term hormonal balance, healthy fat burning, and the best symphony for your cells.

▶ Keep troubleshooting the most common issues in order to solidify the progress you've achieved with four-week Gottfried Protocol pulse.

▶ Remember that you gained weight gradually, and you will lose weight gradually. Go slow with Transition. Keep your eyes focused on long-term weight loss and maintenance.

▶ If you need ongoing support or a daily check-in, return to Chapters 5 and 6, and this chapter. Reread them as often as necessary.

▶ The Gottfried Protocol is not just another diet. It's a tool that allows you to get to know yourself on a deeper level, hormones and all, if you will allow it. It will teach you so much about how your food talks to your hormones, and vice versa. This increased self-awareness, intimacy, and knowledge will serve you for the years and decades to come.

# 8

## INTEGRATION

Done! *Hurray!* In just over four weeks, you solved an enormous problem, one you may not have even known you had. You changed the food on your plate, changed the hormones in your tissues, and as a result, changed your life for the better. I am delighted because the investment you've made in your hormonal symphony will pay dividends for the rest of your life. Regardless of the symptoms you had when you first started this program — crossing a line with your weight, energy, infertility, stubborn belly fat, prediabetes, hot flashes, night sweats, moodiness, anxiety, insomnia, poor stamina — you can now go forward with knowing how foods impact your hormones and body. Consequently, you are now experiencing the benefits of a well-tuned orchestra and improved metabolic flexibility.

Now it's time to create a plan for the rest of your life that integrates hormonal balance. I'm here to cheer you on and provide guidance. I've learned over the years that there's no magic formula that keeps your weight exactly where you want it. Instead, it's the repetition of the little steps provided in this book that add up over time to major transformation. Commit to those steps, because small steps taken consistently are the most impactful. Repeat the Gottfried Protocol if and when symptoms of hormone imbalance recur (refer to pages 26–28 for the questionnaires), when you begin having trouble again with sugar cravings, or when you gain 5 pounds.

As you now know, the goal is metabolic flexibility, the healthy metabolic state in which the body shifts efficiently between the two main fuels: glucose and fat. When you perform intermittent fasting or restrict carbs, your body burns fat. When you eat more than your personal carb limit (defined in Chapter 7), your body burns glucose, setting up cravings for more and triggering fat storage. Insulin runs the show, but now that insulin is in a more balanced state, you can shift easily and rapidly, depending on which fuel is available and appropriate. When insulin is in the healthy range after completion of the Gottfried Protocol, the body can more easily switch between fat and glucose as fuel. I'll repeat: *the point of it all is metabolic flexibility.*

You may have been stuck before the Gottfried Protocol in a pattern of glucose burning from eating sugar or excess carbs, elevated insulin, and even insulin block. Over time, that can lead to other hormone imbalances and serious health problems, as we've discussed.

When food and hormones are out of whack, life is tough, even cruel and inhumane. It can turn us into numbed-out automatons going through the motions of daily experience. It can make us vulnerable to disease. That's especially true during a time of crisis. It can make challenging times feel daunting and frightening, or you may feel nothing at all. Maybe you've experienced significant grief. Maybe you got sick during the pandemic, or faced a different harrowing medical diagnosis. Maybe you gained the "quarantine 15" or have put on weight because of a stressful job. Maybe you lost someone you love, or a job. Taking a prescription pill may seem like the right answer, or at least an easy one.

Here's what I can tell you after a few decades of studying how pharmaceuticals compare to lifestyle changes: lifestyle changes are more effective than almost any prescription. The trick is making sure your values are in the right place, and being resolute about what is truly important to you. No more self-sabotage or internal debates, because you have the deciding vote with your next set of choices, from what's in your grocery cart to what's on your plate. When you can clearly state your values, your behavior aligns with them. The process becomes simple and empowering.

Remember what matters to you

In this final chapter, I want to take a moment to connect to your own desire for change. It's like an internal compass, pointing you toward your next actions, connections with people and places and ideas, and personal codes of conduct. That compelling desire or drive can only come from you. As you consider your desire to improve your metabolic health, I want to praise your success so far and accept any of your weaknesses, false starts, backsliding, or plateaus — all in an atmosphere of collaboration rather than confrontation, judgment, or belittlement.

By this point in *Women, Food, and Hormones,* you have a good sense of your priorities and values regarding food, hormones, and health. You know what your ideal fat mass and weight should be, and how you want your clothes to look and feel. Let's make these ideas more explicit and integrate them more thoroughly into our lives. Why? Because when you take the ambiguity out of what you value most and act in accordance with those values, life becomes simpler, more fun, and definitely more fulfilling. Trust me, life in congruence with your highest values is more like vacation. You are pulled forward by a strong, undeniable vision for yourself. Life is less about control, or the illusion of control that many of us use to cope with fear. Do you ever feel like weight loss is a matter of control? It's not. That's an illusion. Fear and control are not effective for long-term weight loss and health. Instead, long-term success is about valuing your metabolic hormones, metabolic flexibility, and health above all else, and eating in a way that is congruent with your values.

Revisit the personal value statement you wrote back in Chapter 5. Just as your metabolotype may change from apple to pear (or maybe even to celery!), your value statement may evolve to integrate fresh ideas and insights based on your experience. See if your personal value statement needs any editing. (If you skipped the exercise the first time, no problem — go back to Chapter 5 and write it for the first time. It can still be a compass going forward to help you maintain progress.) You may want to amend it by adding certain numbers, like the maximum weight you will allow before repeating the Gottfried Protocol or the minimum muscle mass you envision for yourself as you age.

## IT'S NEVER TOO LATE TO BALANCE YOUR HORMONES

At the beginning of the book, I explained that it's never too late to get your metabolic hormones in order. You now have that enviable clean slate — you are in hormonal homeostasis. While following the Gottfried Protocol, you invested in detoxification, so your liver is no longer maxed out. You can easily fast and heal your body with fourteen to sixteen hours of metabolic rest to induce gentle ketosis. Hopefully, I've empowered you to apply what you know about the food-hormone connection so that you can solve or avoid the problems that are so prevalent in women after age thirty-five, from insulin resistance to diabetes, breast cancer, and heart disease.

You are not stuck with the hormones that you have, even if your doctor has dismissed your concerns or told you there's nothing you can do. The endocrine system, like all parts of the body, is malleable: it can keep growing, learning, storing new memories, and changing itself and the function of the body, often regardless of age and previous issues. You can always get the orchestra back on track. That's the promise and benefit of precision medicine. You want to keep your endocrine system interacting with your inner and outer world, as well as your gastrointestinal, neurological, and immune systems. You want to create balance across the cohesive whole of your body, and food is the great integrator. This level of attention to your food and hormones will keep you in a sound body and mind for years to come.

# MAINTAINING
# A BALANCED YOU

Your task going forward is to keep up the measurement — that is, the regular assessment of your weight, waist and hip measurements, and maybe your fat mass. Decide now, and add to your personal value statement this new line in the sand. If you cross that line because of a cheat day or a birthday celebration, do another pulse of the Gottfried Protocol for one to four weeks. For example, after vacation, I will sometimes follow Implementation for one week to get back on track. Or maybe you have a special event that's six weeks away — you could follow the program for the length of time that you need. However, I do not recommend staying in ketosis for longer than six months because of the limited safety data, particularly for women.

Pick your favorite meals from the past few weeks and make them part of your regular repertoire. Keep working your favorite practice and let it work you.

No doubt you will encounter challenges. Challenges are inevitable, but hormone imbalances are not. Build your resilience: continue feeding your healthy gut microbes by eating plants — and a lot of them, a pound per day. Keep monitoring your blood sugar and ketones after you complete the Gottfried Protocol, maybe every other day for a few weeks, and then once per week if you're stable and in the target zones. Maintain or grow your lean body mass by tracking it at least every quarter or yearly (more often if you are gaining weight) and by performing the exercise combination (two-thirds weight lifting to one-third cardio) that's been shown to be best for cardiovascular health. Sweat more: walk in the forest, practice yoga, or visit a sauna. Cultivate friendships with people who eat mindfully, so you can upgrade your habits and health span together.

You've already made great strides in balancing your hormones; now you want to maintain your progress. Over time, the commitment you make to your favorite Gottfried Protocol practices will aggregate into a habit, and eventually, a sense of integrity and freedom.

We started this book with the analogy of a cool summer breeze for food-based hormonal balance. My hope is that this final chapter adds further motivation, like the wind at your strong back as you move forward toward health and healing. Over the years, I've learned that staying motivated is a process. The weight loss, clarity, peace, equanimity, happiness, and mental focus of the Gottfried Protocol will energize you and keep you motivated, even more so than when you began, if you allow it.

## LIVE YOUR VALUES

When it comes to hormones and body mass, I know what I want. I want to be that woman with sparkling eyes and effusive energy who is changing the conversation about hormones, who is a champion of others, and who practices what she preaches in a loop of integrity. I want to continue to be a leader in the new paradigm of medicine, which includes taking inventory of implicit bias, racial disparities, and health inequities, and promoting anti-racist policy and policy makers. Privately, I want to be emotionally connected with my family and friends, not distracted by thoughts of my thighs or bathroom scale or what to wear. I can't be whole if I'm thinking about whether I have a thigh gap. I want to nurture others. My values are a compass for who I want to be in the world and how I integrate research, studying, synthesis, writing, and teaching. This particular combination of values and roles nourish me, cell to soul.

James Baldwin, the American novelist, playwright, essayist, poet, and activist, wrote the following words: "I have always been struck, in America, by an emotional poverty so bottomless, and a terror of human life, of human touch, so deep that virtually no American appears able to achieve any viable, organic connection between his public stance and his private life." I agree. That's why we need to reach beyond the boundaries of our lives and get very intentional about our highest values and how they can map our life roles. And I hope that includes your unique biology as a woman, particularly your hormones.

Now it's your turn. How can you continue to refine your values and live in accordance with them, so that you avoid emotional poverty? This condition disrupts hormones in a way that food may not help. On the other hand, I've learned recently from a friend that the voids we experience in life can point to our most essential values. Whatever is missing, such as emotional nurturing of ourselves and others, can direct us to the complementary value that creates fulfillment. Personally, I recently left a job because it restricted my freedom to teach the content that matters most to me and also took me away from my family. It showed me how highly I value freedom, autonomy, and family life. Voids create values. What voids are you experiencing? Consider health, body size, your emotional life, your sense of security, the congruence between your public life and private life. Balance requires many inputs—and a prescription for the rest of your life to keep your head, heart, and hormones in balance.

## PLEASE HELP
## SPREAD THE WORD

Lifestyle choices, starting with food, play a huge role in hormonal health, and by extension, a person's total health. Together we need to raise the bar. We have a long way to go—please help spread the message by talking to your doctor and other health-care professionals about the topics in this book and the evidence-based Gottfried Protocol.

Tell your loved ones, especially your mothers, sisters, and daughters, that there is another way to handle the symptoms of hormonal craziness, fat accumulation, and weight gain. Chat with your friends and hair stylist about what you discovered about your own body while following these tenets. In many ways, you are your own best doctor. Share your story of challenge and success with me and others on social media. Help me spread the word. Serving others is good for the hormones. Please help me get the best information out to people who still suffer and desire change.

## CLOSURE

For most of you, the Gottfried Protocol will provide a food-hormone framework that will allow you to reclaim your health and body, making big significant progress over four weeks.

Even though hormones can sometimes be vulnerable, prone to being pulled out of balance by modern lifestyle choices and exposures, the Gottfried Protocol will help you live in a happy, energized, and high-performance state in which food and hormones act as allies. That means there are ongoing, rich, deep conversations occurring between food, metabolic hormones, gut health (including the gut lining, the liver, the microbiome and its microbiota, and the immune system), heart and vascular system health, brain health, mitochondrial health, and fat (subcutaneous and visceral). Without those conversations, we can too easily fall back to the default setting, which we don't want. Avoid it.

Remember too that you've now got a comprehensive food plan in your back pocket — not a restrictive, short-term means to an end but a personalized dietary regimen that you've just tested on yourself. You also launched important daily habits that will help you govern life — in short, the broader precision-medicine protocol that will keep your hormones in homeostasis for the win. All of these new skills and habits, combined with what you've learned by following the Gottfried Protocol, provides closure on past dysfunction and new data to support a fresh start.

Lifestyle medicine is the most effective solution for the hormone dysfunction that we may face as women. Let your lifestyle choices lift you up rather than take you down. We find our own way amid the noise of the diet culture and the anti-diet culture. Ultimately, we get to make a decision about what to do with our food and our bodies. I support you in your decisions. You can get to a place of peace with your hormones and weight while still taking steps to become the healthiest possible version of yourself. Remember, your hormones are an orchestra, and there are no solo acts. There is only an integrated whole.

Finally, I hope you go beyond fixing your metabolic hormones to create a balanced, soulful existence. By creating balance between the sympathetic (fight-flight-freeze) and parasympathetic (rest-and-digest) nervous systems, the hypothalamic-pituitary-adrenal axis, and the endocrine glands, and by favoring positive thoughts and feelings about the body — you restore homeostasis. The only way to achieve it that I know of is with comprehensive lifestyle medicine, not the next prescription pill. It's the small daily choices that will influence your ability to return to balance. Lifestyle factors powerfully affect hormones, and vice versa. Leverage the malleability of your endocrine system and become stronger at the broken places. Your body will be at one with itself. You will get healthier and maybe reverse disease. Your body will learn to rewire itself to serve you and your highest values.

# 9

---

# RECIPES AND
# MEAL PLANS

Now for the fun — and delicious — part! In this chapter, you will find my favorite recipes and meals, which will set you up for success on the Gottfried Protocol. The emphasis is on real whole foods and generous portions of healthy fats in order to restore hormone levels to optimal ranges. Whenever possible, use organic ingredients.

Small amounts of sea salt or kosher salt are suggested as seasoning while in ketosis, as long as you are avoiding processed food that is high in sodium and do not have a condition that warrants sodium restriction (examples include salt-sensitive high blood pressure, impaired kidney function, and increased calcium losses in the urine, but check with your doctor if you are unsure). When you restrict carbohydrates, your body excretes excess fluid, and sodium leaves with it. To make sure you have sufficient sodium levels, sprinkle a little sea salt (approximately ⅛ teaspoon) on your food.

As you will find, I've learned how to modify many popular dishes to make them keto-friendly, so you won't feel deprived or miss your favorite flavors and meals. You can see what I've done and then apply the same process to your most beloved meals.

# SHAKES

I make a shake most mornings after a fourteen- to sixteen-hour fast and a workout (I exercise in a fasted state). My typical workout is two-thirds heavy weights and one-third cardio, but sometimes it's just slow-flow or restorative yoga. Consuming a functional shake is a great way to break a fast with dense nutrients, sufficient protein, and a small amount of carbs to restore the body. These are my favorite Gottfried Protocol shakes, but honestly, there is an infinite number of combinations that you can make from the following recipes, which are merely guides. The first recipe is a template that you can alter to suit your particular tastes and hormone-based requirements. Generally, I aim for 7 to 10 net carbs per meal to stay under my limit of 25 net carbs per day. I recommend using filtered water for all shake recipes. (For more on why filtered water is important, see page 130.)

## The Basic Gottfried Protocol Shake for Ketosis

This great go-to shake is a perfect way to break your fast.

*Serves 1*

**Liquid:** 6–8 ounces filtered water or favorite liquid (such as unsweetened almond, coconut, or cashew milk)

**Vegetables:** ½–1 cup kale, spinach, mixed greens, and/ or 1 scoop Reset360 Super Greens or another organic greens powder

**Shake powder (optional):** 1–2 scoops of a shake powder that provides a ketogenic ratio of 1:1 or better.

**Fat:** ¼ of an avocado, 1–3 tablespoons flaxseed, 1–3 tablespoons soaked chia seeds (or other nuts or seeds), ½–1 tablespoon medium-chain triglyceride (MCT) oil or avocado oil, nut butters, or cacao nibs

**Boosters:** 1–2 scoops supplemental fiber such as Reset360

Daily Fiber or another source of fiber, spirulina or chlorella, dark cacao powder, or cinnamon

**Ice:** 6+ ice cubes

1. In the jar of a high-speed blender, combine ingredients and whip to desired consistency.

## Creamy Green Chia Shake

I like to keep extra greens stacked in glass containers in my freezer so I can easily add them to shakes as desired. This shake is a delicious and nutritious way to get extra greens into your diet. Note that I soak the chia seeds in the morning before my workout, so there is plenty of time for the soluble fiber to soak up to ten to twelve times its weight in water, creating a gel-like consistency that makes the shake creamier. Drinking a shake containing this chia water increases satiety and can help with rebalancing hormones.

*Serves 1*

4 ounces filtered water

2–3 tablespoons chia seeds, depending on desired thickness

2–3 ounces frozen kale

⅓–¼ of an avocado, pit and skin removed

½ cup unsweetened coconut milk (or other unsweetened nut milk)

1 scoop or ½ serving of Reset360 Keto Thrive powder in vanilla

½–1 tablespoon MCT oil

6+ ice cubes

Optional: 1 scoop organic greens powder

Optional: 1–2 scoops supplemental prebiotic fiber

1. In the jar of a high-speed blender, soak chia seeds in filtered water for about 20 minutes before adding other ingredients. Whip to desired consistency.

## Pumpkin Spice Shake

Fresh pumpkin has more carbs than several other vegetables, but it provides many important nutrients, including vitamin A, lutein, and zeaxanthin, all of which may help protect your eyesight. For this recipe, you can roast a small (4–6 pound) pumpkin in the oven at 400 degrees F for about 30 to 45 minutes. Split the pumpkin in half and sprinkle with sea salt. Allow to cool, then store the pumpkin in the refrigerator for up to three days or in the freezer for up to three months.

*Serves 1*

> 4–6 ounces filtered water
> ¼ cup pumpkin puree
> ½ teaspoon cinnamon
> ½ teaspoon allspice
> ½ teaspoon nutmeg
> ¼ teaspoon cloves
> Tiny peel of fresh ginger
> ½ cup unsweetened coconut milk (or other unsweetened nut milk)
> 1–2 scoops of a ketogenic shake powder in vanilla
> ½–1 tablespoon MCT oil
> 6+ ice cubes
> Optional: 1–2 scoops supplemental prebiotic fiber

1. In the jar of a high-speed blender, combine ingredients and whip to desired consistency.

# Post-Workout Shake

I started using cranberries in my shakes during the COVID-19 pandemic when all the other frozen fruit was sold out. Turns out cranberries tend to be neglected, but they are a nutrient powerhouse, with only 4 net carbs per ½ cup. They add tartness and color to a shake, and it's a good idea to aim for a variety of colors in your diet to help support immune resilience. Research shows that brightly colored vegetables and fruits are superior to most supplements in modulating immune function.

*Serves 1*

> ¼–½ cup cranberries
> ½ cup unsweetened coconut milk (or other unsweetened nut milk)
> 1 scoop or ½ serving ketogenic shake powder in vanilla
> ½–1 tablespoon MCT oil
> Handful of nuts (such as macadamia nuts, or others listed on page 119, no more than 28 grams)
> 6+ ice cubes
> Optional: 1-2 scoops supplemental prebiotic fiber

1. Place all ingredients in the jar of a high-speed blender and whip to desired consistency.

## Iced Coffee Collagen Shake

This shake is a great way to get going in the morning — even when made with decaffeinated coffee. Think of it as a more nutritious version of a latte.

*Serves 1*

> 4 ounces unsweetened coffee or decaffeinated coffee, frozen into cubes
> ¼–⅓ of an avocado, pit and skin removed
> 1 cup unsweetened coconut milk (or other unsweetened nut milk)
> 1 scoop or serving of collagen or ketogenic shake powder in vanilla
> ½ teaspoon Ceylon cinnamon
> ½–1 tablespoon MCT oil
> Handful of nuts (such as macadamia nuts, or others listed on page 119, no more than 28–30 grams)
> 6+ ice cubes
> Optional: 1–2 scoops supplemental prebiotic fiber

1. Place all ingredients in the jar of a high-speed blender and whip to desired consistency.

## Almond Butter–Cacao Nib Shake

This shake is like a liquid version of chocolate-almond bark.

*Serves 1*

> 6 ounces unsweetened almond milk
> 2 tablespoons chia seeds
> 1–2 scoops ketogenic shake powder
> 1–2 tablespoons almond butter
> ½–1 tablespoon MCT oil
> Handful of nuts (such as macadamia nuts, or others listed on page 119, no more than 28–30 grams)
> 6+ ice cubes

Optional: 1–2 scoops supplemental prebiotic fiber
Optional: top with chopped almonds (1 teaspoon) and cacao
nibs (1 teaspoon)

1. Soak chia seeds in almond milk for 20 minutes. Place seeds, milk, and remaining ingredients in the jar of a high-speed blender and whip to desired consistency.

## Dragon Fruit Shake

I've been experimenting with low-carb fruits like pitaya (dragon fruit). The amount in this shake does not change my blood sugar levels — it represents 5 net carbs.

*Serves 1*

1 cup unsweetened coconut milk (or other unsweetened
nut milk)
2 tablespoons chia seeds
2 scoops ketogenic shake powder in vanilla
1 scoop Reset360 organic greens powder or ½ cup frozen
greens such as spinach or kale
½–1 tablespoon MCT oil
6+ ice cubes
Optional: 50 grams pitaya (dragon fruit) or other low-carb fruit
Optional: 1–2 scoops supplemental prebiotic fiber

1. Soak chia seeds in milk for 5–10 minutes. Place all ingredients in the jar of a high-speed blender and whip to desired consistency.

## Golden Milk Shake

Golden milk, or turmeric milk, is an anti-inflammatory drink that has been part of Indian food culture for many centuries. You will absorb the inflammation-fighting benefits of turmeric more readily if you combine it with fat.

*Serves 1*

> 1 cup unsweetened coconut milk (or other unsweetened nut milk)
> 1 scoop ketogenic shake powder in vanilla
> ½–1 tablespoon MCT oil
> Golden mix: 1 teaspoon turmeric powder, ½ teaspoon Ceylon cinnamon, ½ inch freshly grated ginger root or ½ teaspoon powdered ginger, and ¼ teaspoon ground cardamom
> 6+ ice cubes
> Optional: 1–2 scoops supplemental prebiotic fiber

1. Place all ingredients in the jar of a high-speed blender and whip to desired consistency.

## Dark Chocolate–Sea Salt Shake

For the chocolate lover!

*Serves 1*

> 1 cup filtered water or unsweetened coconut milk (or other unsweetened nut milk)
> Handful of nuts (such as macadamia nuts, or others listed on page 119, no more than 28 grams)
> 2 scoops ketogenic shake powder in chocolate
> 1–2 scoops supplemental prebiotic fiber
> 1 tablespoon flaxseed
> ¼ teaspoon vanilla extract

1 tablespoon MCT oil
6+ ice cubes
Optional: 1–2 scoops supplemental prebiotic fiber
Optional: ⅛ teaspoon of coarse sea salt

1. Place all ingredients except salt in the jar of a high-speed blender and whip to desired consistency. Optional: sprinkle with sea salt.

## Carrot Cake Shake

This recipe is adapted from one created by my friend Kelly LeVeque, a celebrity nutritionist and bestselling author.

*Serves 1*

1 cup unsweetened almond milk
1–2 scoops ketogenic shake powder in vanilla
1 ½ teaspoons ground cinnamon
1 tablespoon almond butter
1 tablespoon flaxseed
½ cup chopped raw carrots (about 4 net carbs)
½ cup frozen riced cauliflower (about 1.5 net carbs)
Optional: handful of spinach

1. Place all ingredients in the jar of a high-speed blender and whip to desired consistency.

## Deep Green Shake

This shake is packed with detoxifying greens.

*Serves 1*

> 1 cup filtered water or unsweetened coconut milk (or other
> unsweetened nut milk)
> ½ cup of frozen dark leafy greens (spinach, kale, or the like)
> Handful of nuts (such as macadamia nuts, or others listed on
> page 119, no more than 28 grams)
> 2 scoops ketogenic shake powder in vanilla
> 1 tablespoon flaxseed
> ½ teaspoon cinnamon
> ¼ teaspoon vanilla extract
> ½–1 tablespoon MCT oil
> 6+ ice cubes
> Optional: 1 scoop organic greens powder
> Optional: 1 teaspoon spirulina
> Optional: 1–2 scoops supplemental prebiotic fiber

1. Place all ingredients in the jar of a high-speed blender and whip to
   desired consistency.

# BREAKFASTS

## Green Egg Scramble

I keep bamboo bags of greens in my freezer to throw into a shake or a sauté. Make your life easier by stocking up with bags of shredded brussels sprouts, spinach, radicchio, kale, and cabbage.

*Serves 1*

> 2 tablespoons extra-virgin olive oil
> 1 cup shredded greens, such as brussels sprouts, spinach, radicchio, kale, or cabbage
> 2 pastured eggs, whisked
> 1–2 tablespoons fresh herbs such as basil, parsley, or thyme
> ¼ of an avocado, peeled and chopped

1. Sauté greens in olive oil over medium heat until softened. Place bed of greens on a plate. Scramble eggs in remaining oil; add herbs after eggs are set. Top greens with eggs and avocado, and serve immediately.

## Avo Toast

Creamy and satisfying avocado smashed onto well-toasted keto bread is a divine quick meal. I make it by first spreading extra-virgin olive oil and peeled, smashed garlic onto the toast before adding the mashed avo, but there are endless variations.

*Serves 1*

> 1 piece keto bread (about 4 net carbs) – see Tahini Bread recipe (page 206) and Resources
> 1 garlic clove, peeled and crushed
> 1 tablespoon extra-virgin olive oil
> ¼ of an avocado, pit and skin removed
> Fresh lemon juice
> Sea salt
> Optional toppers: chopped herbs (cilantro, dill, parsley), chopped radish, sliced tomato, Pesto (see recipe on page 223), chimichurri, a poached or fried pastured egg, pickled red onion, seeds (pumpkin, sunflower), red pepper flakes

1. Toast bread. Rub the garlic clove on bread, and drizzle with olive oil. Mash avocado in a bowl and spread onto toast. Top with lemon juice and sea salt, to taste. If desired, add another optional ingredient.

# Coffee Cake

I love this bread! You have to commit to taking only one serving — the aroma while it's baking is very tempting. I find that certain sugar substitutes like stevia tend to make me overeat, so I measure my serving and then walk away from the rest of the loaf. Note that I developed this recipe when I was deeply into ketosis. If you have taste buds trained to a crappy carb diet, this keto coffee cake may not taste right to you. But if you're in ketosis, it will taste divine. The flax meal, rich in omega-3s, will help balance your omegas.

*Serves 12 to 15*

> 1 cup filtered water
> ½ cup flax meal
> ½ cup coconut flour (can substitute almond flour)
> ½ teaspoon fine Himalayan pink salt
> 1 teaspoon baking soda
> ½ cup grass-fed butter, plus more to grease the pan (can substitute ghee or coconut oil)
> 1 teaspoon almond extract
> 1 teaspoon ground cinnamon
> 3 pastured eggs
> 1 tablespoon apple cider vinegar
> 3-4 drops liquid stevia (use plain, or consider English toffee flavor)
> ⅓ cup stevia chocolate chips (total 3 net carbs)
> Optional: fresh lemon zest

1. Preheat oven to 350 degrees F. Grease a loaf pan with butter, ghee, or coconut oil.
2. Combine water with flax meal in a small bowl and set aside.
3. In a medium bowl, whisk or sift together coconut flour, salt, and baking soda. Whisk in melted butter, then add eggs and moistened flax mixture. Mix in vinegar, stevia, and chocolate chips. Add lemon zest, if desired, to taste.
4. Place mixture in the greased loaf pan and bake for 40–45 minutes, until the top is browned. Let loaf cool on a rack for 15–30 minutes. To serve, cut into 12 to 15 slices. Store in the refrigerator or freezer.

## Tahini Bread

Tahini (sesame paste) is an excellent choice on the Gottfried Protocol because the macronutrient ratio of fat, protein, and carbs is 76:10:14. Tahini is low in net carbs (about 1.8 net carbs per tablespoon).

*Makes 1 loaf*

> 1 ½ cups tahini
> 4 eggs
> 1 ½ tablespoons apple cider vinegar
> ¾ teaspoon baking soda
> ½ teaspoon salt
> 1 tablespoon sunflower seeds, plus 1 teaspoon for topping
> 1 tablespoon sesame seeds, plus 1 teaspoon for topping
> 1 tablespoon chia seeds, plus 1 teaspoon for topping
> 1 tablespoon pumpkin seeds, plus 1 teaspoon for topping

1. Preheat oven to 350 degrees F, and line a loaf pan with parchment paper.
2. Mix all ingredients until well combined and pour into prepared pan.
3. Sprinkle with reserved teaspoon of each seed, and bake until loaf is slightly brown on top, and firm.

*Courtesy of Nathalie Hadi*

# Frittata with Spinach, Eggplant, and Pine Nuts

I cook this frittata in a cast iron pan to get a small dose of iron along with the stellar amino acid profile of pastured eggs. If you eat dairy-free, you can make this without the heavy cream.

*Serves 4*

> 1 cup Japanese eggplant, cut into ½-inch rounds and then into
>   ½-inch cubes
> Sea salt
> 2 tablespoons extra-virgin olive oil
> 1 cup spinach
> 6–8 pastured eggs
> ¼ cup heavy cream
> 2 tablespoons parsley, chopped
> 2 tablespoons pine nuts, toasted

1. Preheat oven to 350 degrees F. Sprinkle eggplant with sea salt. Sauté eggplant in olive oil over medium heat (don't let it smoke) for about 15 minutes. Add spinach and sauté for 1 more minute. Whisk eggs with heavy cream and pour into pan. Place pan in oven and bake for 20 minutes or until eggs are set. Top with parsley and toasted pine nuts.

# Shakshuka

This Middle Eastern dish, pronounced "shahk-shoo-kah," is traditionally served for breakfast, but you can eat it anytime. It can be served
with a small amount of yogurt, kefir, or tahini, which is the lowest in net
carbs. Traditionally, shakshuka contains tomato paste, but I removed it
because of its sugar content.

*Serves 2 to 4*

> 2 tablespoons grape-seed oil
> 1 large yellow onion, chopped
> 1 red or green bell pepper, chopped
> 1 small hot pepper, deseeded and chopped
> 4 garlic cloves, smashed and chopped
> 2–3 cups ripe tomatoes, chopped
> 2 teaspoons cumin
> 1 teaspoon salt
> 1 teaspoon ground pepper
> 2 cups spinach
> 4 large pastured eggs
> Optional: ½ cup feta cheese
> Optional: ¼ cup fresh parsley, chopped

1. In a large deep pan, heat the oil over medium heat and sauté the
   onions until brown. Add the peppers and garlic. Cook for about 5
   minutes until soft, then add the tomatoes, cumin, salt, and pepper.
   Cover and cook on low heat for another 5 to 10 minutes, stirring often.
2. Add the spinach, and let the vegetables simmer for another 10 to
   15 minutes until you've made a thick sauce. Feel free to taste and
   adjust the seasonings.
3. Once the sauce has thickened, make four small wells in it, in the
   pan. Carefully crack each egg and place one into each of the wells.
   (It's easier if you crack each egg individually into a glass and gently
   pour it into the sauce.) Make sure that the yolks do not break. The
   egg whites should spread out over the sauce; use a fork to swirl the
   whites if needed.
4. Once you've added all the eggs, cover the shakshuka and heat for 5
   to 10 minutes, until the egg whites have cooked. The yolks should

remain slightly soft. Remove from the stove and top, if desired, with feta and fresh parsley. Enjoy this dish while it's hot!

*Adapted from* Brain Body Diet *by Sara Gottfried, MD*

## Egg-Avocado Bake

Avocados are the quintessential ketogenic plant-based food. Halved avocados are a great container for other nutrient-dense foods like an egg or crabmeat. Avocados come in many sizes, so you can scale the recipe for the size of the freshest avocados you can find and, as we discussed earlier, take care not to eat too much avocado each day. Pro tip: put a couple of drops of hot sauce or whatever condiment you like in the hole before you add the egg.

*Serves 2 people per avocado*

> Avocados, halved, pit and skin removed
> Eggs (1 egg per avocado half, meaning 2 per whole avocado)
> Optional: hot sauce, Pesto (see recipe on page 223), chimichurri
> Salt and pepper to taste
> Optional: cilantro, scallions, hot chilies, greens as toppings

1. Scoop out some of the flesh (about 1 tablespoon) of an avocado half, so there is a hole big enough for an egg. Repeat with remaining avocado halves.
2. Put the avocado halves in a small baking dish. You want them to be snug, so they don't tip over. It helps to nestle the avocados in pie weights, dried beans, or coarse salt to keep them standing up straight. Crack one egg at a time into a small ramekin or glass. Slide the egg carefully into the hole of an avocado half; repeat for each half. Season avocado halves with salt and pepper, and drizzle any desired condiments over them. I like to use a little Pesto or chimichurri here. Bake at 450 degrees F for 10 to 12 minutes, or until egg whites are set but the yolks are still a little runny.
3. Douse with greens or other toppings (cilantro, scallions, and hot chilies are all delicious options!).

*Adapted from* Younger *by Sara Gottfried, MD*

# SALADS

## Basic Green Salad

When you make salads, rotate the greens — romaine, red romaine, butterhead, oakleaf, red Lolla Rossa, mesclun, endive, radicchio, spinach, kale, watercress, cabbage, Swiss chard, collard greens, and so on — from day to day. Add any available raw or steamed vegetables, including bell peppers, broccoli, or cauliflower, for example. We know that extra-virgin olive oil is very heart-healthy, so think of salads as a prebiotic vehicle for it. I aim for 4 to 5 tablespoons of extra-virgin olive oil per day — on salads, steamed vegetables, keto bread, and shirataki noodles.

*Serves 2 to 4*

1 tablespoon shallot, peeled and chopped
1 tablespoon red wine vinegar (or another no- or low-
   carbohydrate vinegar like Champagne vinegar or apple
   cider vinegar)
2 cups torn or chopped greens, such as romaine or
   butter lettuce
1 cucumber, chopped (I do not peel if organic)
½ cup bell pepper, sliced
½ cup broccoli sprouts (or any type of sprouts: alfalfa,
   sunflower, mung bean, radish, cress, fenugreek, or the like)
¼ cup carrots, grated
½ cup cherry tomatoes, sliced in half
2–3 tablespoons extra-virgin olive oil
1 tablespoon sunflower seeds
2 tablespoons fresh thyme, chopped
Optional: add ¼ cup grated cheese (such as Parmesan or
   Asiago, or vegan cheese), another healthy protein (such as
   nuts, shrimp, wild salmon), or a combination

1. In a small bowl, soak chopped shallots in red wine vinegar. In a large bowl, combine all the other vegetables.
2. Blend vinegar and shallots with olive oil. Toss this dressing with vegetables, coating them well. Top with sunflower seeds, fresh thyme, and any optional additions.


## Little Gem Salad

Little Gem lettuce has a flavor somewhere between that of romaine and butter lettuce. If you can't find this variety, use half of a heart of romaine instead.

*Serves 2 to 4*

2 cups Little Gem lettuce, torn
½ cup jicama, sliced
¼ cup red onion, sliced
¼ cup poblano chili pepper, chopped
½ of an avocado, halved, pitted, peeled, and sliced
1–2 tablespoons almonds, chopped
2 tablespoons extra-virgin olive oil
1 tablespoon Champagne vinegar
2 tablespoons pumpkin seeds
2 tablespoons cilantro, chopped
Optional: small amount of queso fresca (literally "fresh cheese," usually a mixture of cow and goat cheese), such as cotija or Oaxacan cheese
Optional: moderate amount of protein (2–3 ounces), such as a chicken thigh or drumstick, salmon, low-mercury tuna, or shrimp

1. In a large bowl, combine all ingredients through almonds. Separately, combine olive oil and Champagne vinegar, then drizzle on top of salad, and toss. Top with pumpkin seeds, cilantro, and optional protein.

## Chopped Greens and Marcona Salad

The Marcona almond, known as the "queen of almonds," is imported from Spain. These almonds are shorter and rounder than the California variety. I buy them blanched, roasted in olive oil, and sprinkled with sea salt from the grocery store or online.

*Serves 2 to 4*

> 2 cups greens (such as romaine, mesclun, endive, radicchio, spinach, kale, or the like), chopped
> ½ cup jicama, chopped
> ¼ cup Manchego cheese, chopped
> 2–3 tablespoons Marcona almonds, chopped
> 2–3 tablespoons extra-virgin olive oil
> 1 tablespoon Champagne vinegar (or red or white wine vinegar, or apple cider vinegar)

1. Combine all ingredients through almonds. Whisk olive oil and Champagne vinegar, and toss with salad.

## Tea Leaf Salad

You can purchase organic laphet fermented tea leaves online or at some grocery stores. Or just omit them from the recipe.

*Serves 2 to 4*

> 1 cup romaine lettuce, chopped
> 1 cup green or purple cabbage, chopped
> ½ cup cherry tomatoes, sliced in half
> 1 red bell pepper, sliced
> Tea Leaf Dressing (recipe follows)
> 1–2 tablespoons sunflower seeds
> 1–2 tablespoons sesame seeds
> Optional: peanuts, cooked yellow split peas

1. Place the romaine lettuce in a shallow bowl and top with vegetables. Toss with Tea Leaf Dressing, then top with sunflower and sesame seeds.

## Tea Leaf Dressing

> ¼ cup white vinegar
> ¼ cup loose green-tea leaves (such as sencha) or laphet fermented tea leaves, packed in olive oil
> ¼ cup organic sesame oil
> ¼ cup avocado oil
> ½ tablespoon fish sauce
> Juice of ½ lemon
> 1 tablespoon fresh ginger, minced
> 1 garlic clove, smashed and minced

1. Add ingredients to the jar of a high-speed blender and whip until smooth.

# Crispy Cucumber Salad with Tahini Dressing

Kohlrabi, or German turnip, is another cruciferous vegetable that aids in detoxification. It can be eaten raw or lightly cooked.

*Serves 2 to 4*

> 2–4 Kirby, English, or Persian cucumbers, thinly sliced (I do not peel if organic)
> 2 kohlrabies, thinly sliced
> 1 fennel bulb, thinly sliced
> ½ of a jicama, chopped
> ½ cup red onion, finely chopped
> 1 cup fresh cilantro, chopped
> 3–4 tablespoons Tahini Dressing (recipe follows)
> 2 tablespoons pumpkin seeds

1. In a large bowl, combine the cucumber, kohlrabi, fennel, jicama, and onion. Add the cilantro, and toss well with Tahini Dressing. Top with pumpkin seeds.

*Adapted from* Brain Body Diet *by Sara Gottfried, MD*

# Tahini Dressing

Tahini is made from either hulled or unhulled sesame seeds. Unhulled seeds have a more distinct, bitter flavor, whereas hulled seeds are nuttier and make for creamier tahini. Unhulled whole sesame seeds have more calcium, yet hulled seeds are still quite rich in calcium and other nutrients. It's a question of personal preference. You can use this dressing with Crispy Cucumber Salad or as a topping for grilled chicken or roasted vegetables.

> 1 cup 100 percent pure ground tahini (made of sesame
>     seeds only)
> ½ cup filtered water, room temperature or warmed
> ¼ cup extra-virgin olive oil
> ¼–½ cup fresh lemon juice
> 3–4 garlic cloves, smashed and finely chopped
> Dash of salt
> Dash of black pepper

1. Place the ingredients through garlic in a sealable container, and shake well until fully combined. The mixture should turn from a paste into a white sauce. Add more water or lemon juice until the dressing reaches your preferred consistency and flavor. Season with salt and pepper.

*Adapted from* Brain Body Diet *by Sara Gottfried, MD*

## "Taco" Salad

This version of the taco salad is dense with nutrients, without losing the yum factor. The onion in the ground meat and the Pico de Gallo (recipe follows) adds prebiotic fiber to promote healthy microbiota in the gut. I prefer Pico de Gallo to salsa in this salad because it's chunkier, crunchier, and less runny.

*Serves 4 to 6*

> 1 pound of grass-fed, grass-finished ground beef (may
>   substitute pastured ground chicken, turkey, or pork)
> 1 medium yellow onion, chopped
> 1 tablespoon extra-virgin olive oil
> 1 teaspoon ground cumin
> 1–2 heads romaine lettuce, torn into bite-sized pieces
> 1 red cabbage, sliced and diced
> 1 avocado, pitted, peeled, and chopped
> 2 Persian cucumbers, coarsely chopped (I do not peel if
>   organic)
> 8 ounces cheddar cheese, grated (I like raw-milk cheddar,
>   medium sharp; a nondairy cheese can be substituted)
> Pico de Gallo (recipe follows)
> Keto Taco Dressing (recipe follows)
> Optional: ½ cup full-fat sour cream (can substitute
>   crème fraîche or full-fat plain yogurt), fresh herbs,
>   chopped avocado

1. Prepare the meat first. In a medium saucepan, add olive oil and most of the chopped yellow onion (reserve 2 tablespoons for Pico de Gallo). When onion is softened, add ground meat and work with a wooden spoon to break into small crumbles. Cook until meat is brown throughout, then add cumin.
2. Assemble Pico de Gallo.
3. Create a bed of romaine lettuce and red cabbage (about 4–8 ounces per person). Cover with ground meat (3–4 ounces for women, 5–6 ounces for men). Add remaining ingredients in layers; top with grated cheese and, if desired, a dollop of sour cream or other topping option. Add Pico de Gallo and Keto Taco Dressing to taste.

## Pico de Gallo

¼ cup tomatoes, chopped
3 scallions, chopped
Chopped fresh chilies (or ½ teaspoon chipotle powder)
Juice of 1 lime
1 tablespoon chopped fresh cilantro

1. Combine ingredients in a small bowl.

## Keto Taco Dressing

1–2 fresh chipotle peppers or ½ teaspoon chipotle powder
Juice of 1 lemon
2 tablespoons extra-virgin olive oil

1. Whip ingredients in the jar of a high-speed blender until smooth.

## Torn Greens with Ranch Dressing

My family loves to spoon this delicious Ranch Dressing over grilled romaine hearts or use it as a dip for cucumber slices. By the way, why tear salad greens? Because it increases their nutrient density.

*Serves 2 to 4*

> 2–8 cups romaine lettuce, kale, spinach, or other greens, torn
> 1 cup Mayonnaise (recipe follows, or purchase a brand made with avocado oil)
> Ranch Dressing (recipe follows)

## Mayonnaise

> 1 cup avocado oil, extra-virgin olive oil, or a mixture
> 1 yolk from a pastured egg
> 1 tablespoon Dijon mustard
> Juice of ½ lemon
> ½ teaspoon salt

1. Place all ingredients in a narrow container or jar. I use the mixing cup that came with my immersion blender, but a half-pint jar works well too. Place the head of the immersion blender at the bottom of the jar and turn the blender on. The bottom of the jar should quickly emulsify (you'll see it turn white and thick). Slowly move the immersion blender up toward the top of the jar as the mixture emulsifies. If any oil slips back down into the jar, simply move the head of the blender down to mix it in, then continue lifting the blender up toward the surface until all the oil is incorporated and the mixture is thick. This process takes 1 to 2 minutes.
2. This Mayonnaise will keep covered in the refrigerator up to 1 week, depending on the freshness of your egg.

*From* Younger *by Sara Gottfried, MD*

# Ranch Dressing

¼ cup coconut milk
1 teaspoon apple cider vinegar
1 teaspoon onion powder
1 garlic clove, finely minced
1 teaspoon dried dill or 1 tablespoon fresh, minced
2 teaspoons dried parsley or 2 tablespoons fresh, minced
1 tablespoon dried chives or 3 tablespoons fresh, minced
Salt and pepper to taste

1. Add these ingredients to 1 cup of Mayonnaise. Stir until well combined. Add coconut milk as needed to thin the mixture. Season with salt and pepper to taste. Pour the dressing over the torn greens, and toss.
2. Ranch Dressing will keep for 1 week, covered, in the refrigerator. It will thicken as it chills.

*Adapted from* Younger *by Sara Gottfried, MD*

# Seaweed Salad

Seaweed is high in essential minerals, including iodine, calcium, iron, copper, magnesium, manganese, molybdenum, phosphorus, potassium, selenium, vanadium, and zinc. Some seaweed salads that can be bought premade include added sugar or not-so-great oils and vinegars. Here's one that's cleaned up, ready to spruce up your thyroid function.

*Serves 2 to 4*

> 2 ounces dried wakame (or a seaweed mix)
> 1 small daikon radish, julienned
> ½ English cucumber, julienned (I do not peel if organic)
> 1 tablespoon extra-virgin olive oil
> 1 teaspoon sesame oil
> Juice of half a lime or half a lemon
> 2 teaspoons fresh ginger juice
> 1 tablespoon tamari (gluten-free soy sauce)
> 4 tablespoons walnut or avocado oil
> ½ teaspoon stevia, or to taste
> Pinch of sea salt
> Optional: toasted sesame seeds, crushed roasted nori,
>    diced avocado

1. Soak seaweed in cold water for about 5 minutes, until it's rehydrated and no longer tough. Rinse and drain. If there are any large pieces, chop them. Combine the seaweed, daikon, and cucumber in a medium bowl.
2. To make the dressing, mix the remaining ingredients in a small bowl. Add dressing to seaweed mixture, toss, and let sit for a few minutes for the dressing to be absorbed. Add optional toppings if desired, and eat salad with chopsticks.

*Adapted from* Younger *by Sara Gottfried, MD*

# Kale and Caesar Salad with "Raw Parmesan"

A dairy-free version of the classic. If you want to get a jump-start on preparing this salad, make the dressing ahead of time. It will keep for twenty-four hours in the refrigerator.

*Serves 4 to 6*

> 1 bunch lacinato kale
> 2 heads romaine lettuce
> 1 cup cherry tomatoes, halved
> ½ cup cashews, soaked for 2 hours or more
> ¼ cup hemp
> ¼ cup nutritional yeast
> Juice of 2 lemons
> 1 garlic clove, crushed
> ½ teaspoon sea salt or pink Himalayan salt
> ⅓ cup filtered water
> ⅓ cup extra-virgin olive oil
> Optional topping: "Raw Parmesan" (recipe follows)

1. Destem the kale, then finely chop the leaves. Rinse, spin in a salad spinner, then pat dry. Place kale in an extra-large bowl. Tear the romaine into bite-size pieces. Rinse, spin in a salad spinner, then pat dry. Add lettuce to the bowl of kale. You should have roughly 2 to 3 cups of chopped kale and 4 to 6 cups of torn romaine. Fold in cherry tomatoes.
2. To make the dressing, rinse and drain the cashews. In a blender or food processor, combine the cashews and the remaining ingredients. Blend until smooth. Add the dressing to the greens, and toss until coated. If needed, add salt to taste, and toss again. If desired, sprinkle salad with "Raw Parmesan" and serve.

## "Raw Parmesan"

> ½ cup macadamia or cashew nuts, not soaked
> 1 teaspoon nutritional yeast (or more, to taste)
> Optional: pinch of garlic powder

1. Grate the nuts, or process them in a food processor. Add remaining ingredients, and mix or process until combined.

*Adapted from* Younger *by Sara Gottfried, MD*

## Cauliflower Ceviche

Cauliflower may be the most versatile vegetable in the Gottfried Protocol.

*Serves 2 to 4*

> 1 head of cauliflower
> 1 small red onion, diced
> 3 tomatoes, diced
> 2 red chilies, diced
> ½ cup cilantro, chopped
> Juice of 5 lemons
> Sea salt and pepper
> 1 tablespoon extra-virgin olive oil

1. Steam whole cauliflower for 5 minutes. Cut into small pieces.
2. Mix cauliflower, vegetables, and cilantro in a big bowl. Add lemon juice, salt, and pepper to taste, and combine well. Leave in refrigerator to marinate for 30 minutes. Drizzle with olive oil, and serve.

*Adapted from Nathalie Hadi*

# SAUCES AND SALSAS

Keep keto boredom at bay! These sauces and salsas are great to have on hand in the refrigerator, so that you can add zing to your meals, along with healthy extra-virgin olive oil and other phytonutrients.

## Chermoula (Moroccan Green Sauce)

> 2 garlic cloves, peeled and crushed, then chopped
> ¼ cup extra-virgin olive oil
> ¼ cup parsley, chopped
> ½ cup cilantro, chopped
> 1 teaspoon paprika
> ½ teaspoon cumin
> Juice of 1 lemon
> Sea salt to taste

1. Pound garlic with a mortar and pestle. Add herbs and remaining ingredients, then mix well.

## Pesto

I love pesto made with a wide range of greens. Certainly basil and pine nuts are the classic base, but you can use my template in this recipe and apply chard, kale, arugula, and any other greens, and combine them with any of your favorite nuts. Delicious on shirataki noodles or keto toast!

> 2 garlic cloves, peeled, crushed, and chopped
> 2 tablespoons of nuts, such as pine nuts, walnuts, or almonds
> 2 cups greens, such as basil, or kale or chard with stems cut away
> ½ cup Parmigiano-Reggiano, grated
> ¼ cup extra-virgin olive oil

1. Process garlic and nuts in a food processor. Add greens and olive oil, then add cheese last, and process again.

## Pepita Salsa

I love this salsa on flaxseed crackers (available at grocery stores and on-line) or keto bread.

     ½ cup roasted pumpkin seeds
     ½ cup extra-virgin olive oil
     ¼ cup cilantro
     1 tablespoon white wine vinegar

1. Combine ingredients in the jar of a high-speed blender and whip until smooth.

# SOUPS AND BROTHS

## Alkaline Broth with Collagen

Give yourself a nonsurgical facelift with this collagen boost. This broth is delicious to sip, hot or cold, when you feel like you need a little something extra.

*Serves 2 to 12*

> 1–2 cups of three of the following vegetables, roughly chopped: celery, fennel, green beans, zucchini, spinach, kale (destemmed), chard (destemmed), carrots, onion, garlic, cabbage
> ½–1 teaspoon spice (such as cumin or turmeric)
> Filtered water (enough to cover the vegetables)
> Optional: 1 tablespoon powdered collagen protein (Bulletproof and Great Lakes are good brands)

1. Place vegetables and spices in a large soup pot, and cover with filtered water. Bring to a boil, then simmer on low for 30 to 45 minutes. Strain the broth, and set vegetables aside for another use. Whisk in the powdered collagen protein, if using.

*Adapted from* Younger *by Sara Gottfried, MD*

# Avgolemono (Lemon-Chicken Soup with Riced Cauliflower)

In college, avgolemono was my favorite Greek comfort soup. I've adapted this version with riced cauliflower, but I've seen other recipes that use sesame seeds. This recipe has about 5–6 net carbs per serving.

*Serves 4*

> 4 tablespoons extra-virgin olive oil
> 1 yellow onion, finely chopped
> 6 celery stalks, minced
> 3 cups riced cauliflower
> 4 cups Chicken Bone Broth (see recipe on page 227)
> 2 pastured eggs, at room temperature and beaten
> 4 pastured chicken thighs, cooked and shredded
> Juice of 1 lemon
> Salt and pepper to taste
> Optional: lemon zest, chopped parsley

1. In a Dutch oven or stockpot, heat olive oil over medium heat. Stir in onion and celery, and cook until translucent. Add riced cauliflower and Chicken Bone Broth, and stir to combine. Remove soup from heat, and cool for at least 10 minutes.

2. Remove ¼ cup of stock, place in a bowl, and whisk the eggs into it energetically, so that the egg whites do not curdle. Very slowly whisk this egg-stock mixture into the remaining cooled stock. Add chicken, stir, and gently reheat. Season with salt and pepper. Serve immediately, with a squirt of the fresh lemon juice; top with lemon zest and parsley, if using. This soup can be kept in the refrigerator for 3–4 days or stored in the freezer, in an airtight container, for 3 months.

# BONE BROTHS

Bone broth is rich in collagen, a protein needed for healthy skin, teeth, and nails. Your body's production of collagen declines with age, which is why those wrinkles, neck wattles, and weak joint cartilage can catch up with us. For our family, making bone broth is the most convenient way to get collagen into our food plan. If the process sounds disgusting, just start with chicken bones, filtered water, and a slow cooker—the slow cooking breaks the collagen down into gelatin. You'll be amazed. You can use the broth recipes when broth is called for in other dishes in this chapter. Expect cooking your own broth to take several hours. You can also purchase powdered bone broth at the grocery store or online.

## Chicken Bone Broth

*Serves 2 to 12*

> Bones, feet, and neck from 1 chicken
> 2 small onions or shallots, roughly chopped
> 1 head garlic
> 1 teaspoon peppercorns
> 1 or 2 bay leaves
> 2 tablespoons sea salt
> 2 tablespoons apple cider vinegar
> 4 quarts filtered water
> 1 bunch fresh herbs, such as tarragon, per serving

1. Put all the ingredients except the fresh herbs into a large stockpot and let sit for an hour. Bring the broth to a boil, and get rid of any foam that rises to the top. Cook on a very low flame for 8 to 12 hours. Let cool. Separate the meat (if any) from the bones. Strain the broth. Allow to cool, and place in glass jars, leaving 1 to 2 inches of space at the top to prevent breakage of the glass. Keep in the refrigerator for up to 4 days, or freeze.

2. To serve, warm a serving of strained broth to the desired temperature (do not boil). Wash the fresh herbs, and add a large handful for extra minerals and taste.

*Adapted from* Younger *by Sara Gottfried, MD*

## Beef Bone Broth

*Serves 2 to 12*

> 2 pounds (or more) femur bones from grass-fed cattle,
>      or other bones from a healthy source
> Optional: 2 feet from pastured chicken, for extra gelatin
> Filtered water (enough to cover contents)
> 2 tablespoons apple cider vinegar
> 1 onion, roughly chopped
> 2 carrots, roughly chopped
> 2 stalks celery, roughly chopped
> 1 tablespoon or more sea salt
> 1 teaspoon peppercorns
> Optional: additional herbs or spices, to taste
> 2 cloves garlic, roughly chopped
> 1 bunch parsley, roughly chopped

1. If you are using raw bones, especially raw beef bones, it improves flavor to roast them in the oven before making the broth. Place them in a pan, and roast for 30 minutes at 350 degrees F. Then put the bones, including the chicken feet, if using, in a 5-gallon stockpot. Pour the filtered water over the bones, and add the vinegar. Let sit for 20 to 30 minutes. The acid from the vinegar helps make the nutrients in the bones more bioavailable.

2. Add onions, carrots, and celery to the pot. Season with salt, peppercorns, and additional spices or herbs, if using. Bring the broth to a boil. Once it has reached a vigorous boil, reduce heat to a simmer, and keep the broth simmering until it is done.

3. During the first few hours of simmering, remove the impurities that float to the surface. A frothy or foamy layer will form and can

be easily scooped off with a big spoon and thrown away. I typically check the broth every 20 minutes for the first two hours to do this. Bones from grass-fed, healthy animals produce far fewer impurities than bones from conventionally raised animals.

4. During the last 30 minutes, add the garlic and parsley.

5. Remove broth from the heat, and allow it to cool. Strain the broth, using a fine-mesh strainer to remove all the bits of bone and vegetable. Store cooled broth in quart-sized glass jars (leave 1–2 inches of space at the top to prevent breakage of the glass) in the refrigerator for up to four days, or in the freezer to use later.

*Adapted from* Younger *by Sara Gottfried, MD*

## Fish Bone Broth

Bone broth detoxifies and nourishes the kidneys, according to traditional Chinese medicine. Fish stocks made from fish heads have thyroid-strengthening properties. For this recipe, do not use bones from oily fish, such as salmon, because the broth will stink up the whole house! Use only non-oily fish, such as sole, turbot, rockfish, or my favorite, snapper. I use this broth as a base for shirataki noodles and vegetables such as purple cabbage, broccoli, and bell peppers.

*Serves 2 to 12*

> 3 quarts filtered water
> 2 pounds fish heads and bones (fish heads alone will suffice)
> ¼ cup raw, organic apple cider vinegar
> Himalayan or Celtic sea salt to taste

1. Place water and fish heads and bones in a 4-quart stockpot. Stir in vinegar while bringing the water to a gentle boil. As the water rolls and bubbles, skim off any foam that rises to the surface. It is important to do this because the foam contains impurities and off flavors. Reduce heat to a simmer, and cook broth for at least 4 hours but no more than 24. Add salt at the end of cooking, to taste. Cool and then strain the broth into containers for refrigeration. Freeze what you will not use in one week.

# Chicken-Ginger Soup with Cabbage "Pasta"

Get creative by substituting vegetables for pasta. Good candidates include cabbage (as in this recipe), hearts of palm, and spiralized zucchini (also known as zoodles).

*Serves 4*

> 2 tablespoons extra-virgin olive oil (or coconut oil)
> 1-inch piece of fresh ginger (or more, if you like it spicy), washed, peeled, and diced
> 1 medium yellow onion, diced
> 2–4 cloves of garlic, crushed and sliced
> 2 quarts filtered water
> 4 pastured chicken thighs, bone in
> ¼ green cabbage, finely shredded (a chiffonade)
> 2 tablespoons MCT oil
> Sea salt and pepper
> Optional: fresh cilantro or tarragon, torn, as garnish

1. Prepare the base. Heat the olive oil in a large soup pot over medium heat, and add the ginger, onion, and garlic. Cook for 5 minutes, stirring, until onion is translucent. Add water and chicken, and bring to a boil. Continue simmering for 30 minutes or until the chicken is thoroughly cooked.
2. Remove ginger and chicken. Shred the chicken and return it to the soup. Season with salt and pepper to taste.
3. To serve, place a bed of cabbage (about ½ cup) in each bowl. Ladle soup over cabbage. Top with ½ tablespoon of MCT oil and fresh torn herbs, if using.
4. Store soup base in the freezer for up to one month or in the refrigerator for 3–5 days.

# Gazpacho

A refreshing summer soup, made keto with extra-virgin olive oil.

*Serves 4 to 6*

> 2–3 green, red, and yellow peppers, seeded
> 1–2 cucumbers (I do not peel if organic)
> 1 red onion, peeled and diced
> 1 avocado, halved, pitted, peeled, and chopped
> 1 cucumber, diced
> 3 medium heirloom tomatoes, diced
> 2 garlic cloves, smashed and diced
> 2 tablespoons fresh lemon juice
> 2 tablespoons apple cider vinegar
> 2 tablespoons each chopped basil, parsley, and cilantro
> 1 cup extra-virgin olive oil
> Optional: a clump of fresh crabmeat as topping

1. Place peppers and cucumber(s) in the jar of a high-powered blender and puree. In a bowl, combine this mixture with the remaining ingredients, and chill for 3–4 hours. Gazpacho keeps in the fridge for up to 5 days.

## Sorrel Soup

*Easy to Make Vegan or Vegetarian*

*Serves 4, hot or cold*

8 ounces unsalted grass-fed butter

2 yellow onions, diced

4–6 garlic cloves, smashed and diced

10 cups fresh sorrel leaves, rinsed, with stems removed

4 cups Chicken Bone Broth (see recipe on page 227) or
vegetable/vegan broth

1 cup fresh Italian flat-leaf parsley

2 teaspoons grated nutmeg

Pinch of cayenne pepper

Himalayan sea salt and black pepper to taste

1 cup full-fat sour cream or crème fraîche

Optional: fresh chopped chives for garnish

1. Melt the butter in a soup pot over medium heat. Add the onions and garlic and cook, covered, until tender and translucent, about 15 minutes. Add the sorrel, cover, and cook until it is completely wilted, about 5 minutes.

2. Add bone broth, parsley, nutmeg, and cayenne, and bring to boil. Reduce heat, cover, and simmer for 50 minutes. Add salt and pepper to taste.

3. Transfer soup in batches to a blender, and puree until smooth. If serving hot, return soup to pot and heat slowly over low heat, stirring constantly. If serving cold, transfer to a glass or stainless steel bowl, cover, and chill at least 4 hours in the refrigerator. Ladle into bowls and garnish with sour cream or crème fraîche and chives, if using.

# French Onion Soup

A twist on the classic to support the microbiome.

*Serves 4 to 6*

> 1–2 tablespoons grape-seed oil
> 3 large yellow or white onions, quartered and thinly sliced
> 6 cups vegetable broth, or 4 cups filtered water plus 2 cups
>     Chicken Bone Broth (see recipe on page 227)
> 2 cups greens (kale, chard, or spinach), thinly sliced
> 1 bay leaf
> ½ cup fresh thyme, chopped
> Sea salt to taste
> 1 teaspoon fresh ground pepper
> ½ cup grated vegan cashew-nut cheese or nutritional
>     yeast flakes
> ¼ cup green onions, chopped

1. Heat the grape-seed oil in a large pot, and cook the onions until they are soft and browned.
2. Add the broth, greens, and bay leaf. Season soup with thyme, salt, and pepper. Simmer over low heat for 1 hour.
3. To serve, top each bowl of soup with cashew nut cheese or nutritional yeast flakes and green onions.

# Thai Coconut-Chicken Soup (Tom Kha Gai)

*Easy to Make Vegan or Vegetarian*

Kaffir lime leaves are sometimes hard to find. The zest and juice of one lime can be substituted. You can make this soup without chicken, and instead of fish sauce, use vegetarian broth and tamari.

*Serves 6 to 8*

2 stalks lemongrass
1 large piece of Chinese ginger, peeled and chopped
2 cloves garlic
10–12 kaffir lime leaves
2 whole cardamom pods
6 cups Chicken Bone Broth (see recipe on page 227)
1 pound pastured chicken breast or thighs, cut into
    1-inch pieces
1 cup chopped shiitake mushrooms
1 13.5-ounce can unsweetened coconut milk
3 tablespoons fish sauce
Chili oil and cilantro leaves for serving

1. Remove base of lemongrass stalks with a sharp knife, and discard tough outer layer.
2. Chop lemongrass stalks into 2-inch pieces and toss into a blender with the chopped ginger, kaffir lime leaves, and garlic cloves. Pulse a few times until ingredients form a pulp. Add blended ingredients plus 2 cardamom pods to large stockpot over medium-high heat, cooking for 1 to 2 minutes, until fragrant. Add Chicken Bone Broth. Once it's boiling, reduce heat to low and simmer for 20 to 30 minutes, to allow flavors to infuse. Strain the broth through a fine sieve into a large clean pan.
3. Add chicken and mushrooms to broth, and simmer for 20 to 25 minutes, until chicken is cooked through. Remove from heat. Stir in the coconut milk and fish sauce. Garnish with chili oil and fresh cilantro leaves.

# Tofu Masala Soup

This delicious soup contributed to Dr. Anu French's success on the Gottfried Protocol.

*Serves 4*

> 1 tablespoon ghee
> ½ red onion, chopped
> 2 cloves garlic, minced
> 1-inch piece of ginger
> 2 tablespoons olive oil
> 1 cup sliced portabella mushrooms
> ½ bell pepper, chopped
> 1 cup cherry tomatoes, sliced
> ½ teaspoon turmeric powder
> ½ teaspoon garam masala
> 3 cups veggie broth
> 1 cup bok choy, roughly chopped
> 6 ounces extra-firm tofu, cut into cubes
> Salt to taste

1. Add ghee to a large soup pot, and sauté red onions, garlic, and ginger until onions are translucent.
2. Add 1 tablespoon of the olive oil, then the mushrooms, bell pepper, tomatoes, turmeric, and garam masala, and sauté 5 minutes. Add the broth to this mixture and allow to come to a brief boil, then add bok choy and tofu. Add remaining 1 tablespoon olive oil. Add salt to taste. Simmer for another 10 minutes.

*Courtesy of Anu French, MD*

# Creamy Goddess Greens Soup

This soup is delicious hot or cold. Make extra for lunch the next day. Easy to make vegan or vegetarian.

*Serves 4 to 6*

> 2 tablespoons coconut oil
> 3 cups cauliflower florets, chopped
> 6 asparagus spears, chopped
> 2 large shallots, thinly sliced
> 2 cloves garlic, smashed and roughly chopped
> 1 cup arugula
> 1 cup broccoli rabe florets
> ½ cup watercress leaves
> 3 cups organic vegetable or free-range chicken broth
> ¾ cup coconut milk
> 3 tablespoons lemon juice
> ¼ teaspoon cayenne pepper
> 1 teaspoon dried rosemary
> 2 tablespoons extra-virgin olive oil
> Salt and pepper to taste

1. Heat coconut oil in a large soup pot over medium heat. Add cauliflower, asparagus, shallots, and garlic, and cook until cauliflower is tender and shallots are translucent.
2. Reduce heat to low. Stir in arugula, broccoli rabe, and watercress. Keep stirring over low heat until leaves have brightened.
3. Add broth.
4. Working in batches, transfer soup to a blender, and puree until smooth.
5. Return to pot over low heat. Stir in coconut milk, lemon juice, cayenne, rosemary, olive oil, salt, and pepper.

# MAIN DISHES

## Tahini-Sesame Noodles

When I'm on the Gottfried Protocol, one of my favorite swaps for pasta is shirataki noodles, or "miracle noodles," made from konjac root, an excellent source of prebiotic fiber. Konjac root is the source of glucomannan, a type of fiber that has been shown to be associated with weight loss. Konjac grows in Japan, China, and Southeast Asia. *Shirataki* is Japanese for "white waterfall," a reference to the noodles' translucent appearance. It comes in a variety of noodle shapes, from fettuccine to angel hair, and in the shape of grains of rice. (See Resources for the brands that I use.) This calorie-free, carb-free food is 97 percent water and 3 percent glucomannan. It absorbs sauces very well — just be sure to rinse it well in a colander with warm filtered water before using.

*Serves 2*

> 2 tablespoons tahini
> Juice of 1 lemon
> 4 tablespoons MCT oil or extra-virgin olive oil
> 2 teaspoons sesame oil
> 1 tablespoon tamari
> 1 cup of chopped or ribboned vegetables of your choice (I love broccoli, purple cabbage, and zoodles — noodles made from zucchini)
> 1–2 packages of shirataki noodles, fettuccine style, rinsed in warm water

1. Combine tahini with lemon juice, MCT oil (or olive oil), sesame oil, and tamari. Whisk until smooth. In a large bowl, create a bed of shirataki (you don't need to cook them — just rinse in warm water), add the vegetables, and top with the tahini mixture. Toss and serve.

# Kimchi, Shirataki, and Bok Choy Bowl

If you want to avoid cooking with oil, you can steam the vegetables instead of sautéing them and add the olive oil before serving.

*Serves 2*

> 2 tablespoons extra-virgin olive oil
> 14 ounces (2 packages) vermicelli-style shirataki noodles
> 4 cups baby bok choy, thinly sliced
> 2 Japanese eggplants, thinly sliced (about 2 cups)
> 2 tablespoons sesame seeds
> 2 cups greens (kale, chard, or spinach), thinly sliced
> Kimchi to taste
> 1 tablespoon organic sesame oil
> 1–2 tablespoons extra-virgin olive oil

1. Over medium heat, sauté half the shirataki noodles (1 package), baby bok choy, and Japanese eggplant in olive oil (alternatively, you could steam them). Sprinkle with sesame seeds.
2. Assemble all ingredients in a pretty bowl: greens and uncooked shirataki on the bottom, sautéed mixture in the middle, and kimchi on the top. Drizzle with sesame oil and olive oil.

*Adapted from* Brain Body Diet *by Sara Gottfried, MD*

# Vegetable "Fettuccine" Alfredo

The "fettuccine" noodles in this recipe are made of vegetables. Unlike the traditional heavy Alfredo sauce, the one in this recipe relies on Brazil nuts to provide substance and texture. It's fine to vary the amounts of vegetables as you prefer.

*Serves 4*

2 extra-large turnips, spiralized
1 cup carrots, shredded
2 cups lacinato kale, destemmed and shredded
6 tablespoons Brazil nut butter (or ½ cup Brazil nuts)
6 tablespoons water
2 tablespoons apple cider vinegar
2 tablespoons tamari
Sea salt to taste

1. Combine the turnips, carrots, and kale in a large bowl. To make the sauce, blend the rest of the ingredients in the jar of a high-speed blender. Pour about ¼ cup of the sauce over the vegetables, adding more if you need it, to create an even coating. Store the leftover sauce in the refrigerator for up to 3 days.

# Salmon and Avocado Bowl with Miso Dressing

*Serves 4*

> 4 6-ounce salmon fillets (or steelhead trout, which has a
>     similar taste)
> 1 or 2 lemons, sliced in half for rubbing
> Sea salt
> 2 teaspoons fresh lime juice
> 2 teaspoons white miso
> 2 teaspoons filtered water
> ¼ teaspoon freshly ground pepper
> 3 tablespoons extra-virgin olive oil
> 6 cups romaine lettuce, torn
> 1 avocado, peeled and diced
> ¾ cup cucumber, sliced (I don't peel if organic)
> ½ of a red bell pepper, thinly sliced
> ¼ cup walnuts, toasted

1. Preheat the broiler. Place the oven rack about 6 inches from the broiler. Line a baking sheet with foil.
2. Arrange the salmon fillets on the sheet, skin side down. Rub them with lemon and season with sea salt. Broil until the salmon is just cooked through, 7 to 10 minutes (depending on thickness). Remove the skin from each fillet. Chop salmon into generous bite-size pieces.
3. While salmon is cooking, prepare the dressing: In a small bowl, whisk together the lime juice, miso, water, and pepper. While whisking, slowly pour in the extra-virgin olive oil.
4. In a large bowl, combine cooked salmon with lettuce, avocado, cucumber, and red bell pepper, and toss. Divide among four plates. Drizzle 1 tablespoon of the miso dressing over each salad. Top with walnuts and serve.

*Adapted from* Younger *by Sara Gottfried, MD*

## Grilled Salmon Steaks with Lemon-Herb Mojo

Can you tell I love salmon? It's my top choice for resolving inflammation by means of your fork.

*Serves 2*

> 8 ounces salmon steak
> Sea salt and pepper for seasoning
> 1 teaspoon sesame or grapeseed oil
> 1 cup Lemon-Herb Mojo (recipe follows)

1. Preheat oven to 450 degrees F. Season salmon with salt and pepper and place on foil with sesame or grapeseed oil. Bake salmon until cooked through, approximately 12 to 15 minutes. Plate with a generous serving of Lemon-Herb Mojo.

## Lemon-Herb Mojo

This sauce is superb on salads, roasted vegetables, chicken, or fish.

> Juice of 2 lemons
> 3–4 tablespoons avocado oil or extra-virgin olive oil
> 2–3 garlic cloves, roughly chopped
> ½ of a red onion, roughly chopped
> ½ cup fresh cilantro or parsley
> Sea salt to taste

1. Place all the ingredients in a food processor. Pulse to combine until you've created a fragrant, well-blended sauce.

*Adapted from* Brain Body Diet *by Sara Gottfried, MD*

## Halibut with Almond Crust

I love making this dish with halibut from Alaska, where I attended high school. You can substitute salmon or other fish fillets that will hold up to the almond coating.

*Serves 6*

6 halibut fillets, approximately 3 to 6 ounces each
Sea salt and pepper
1 teaspoon grape-seed oil
1 cup chopped blanched almonds
¼ cup chopped fresh parsley
1 tablespoon lemon zest
1 pastured egg, beaten

1. Preheat oven to 400 degrees F. Sprinkle halibut with salt and pepper. Mix almonds, parsley, and lemon zest in a shallow dish. Brush fillets with egg and press into almond mixture to coat.
2. Oil a baking sheet, and place halibut on top. Bake until cooked and crust is brown, about 12 to 15 minutes, depending on the thickness of fillets.

*Adapted from Nathalie Hadi*

# Black Cod with Miso

If you're tired of salmon at this point, consider black cod, also known as sablefish. It has as much omega-3 fat as salmon.

*Serves 2*

> 2 tablespoons regular olive oil (not extra-virgin, which has a
>    lower smoke point)
> ½ cup white miso paste
> 3 tablespoons tamari
> Optional: 1 tablespoon erythritol sweetener or few drops of
>    stevia (optional)
> 1 pound (2 to 4 fillets) black cod
> Avocado oil for pan

1. To make marinade, mix the olive oil, white miso paste, tamari, and sweetener, if using, in a container and set aside. Clean the fillets and pat them dry. Place the fillets in the container, coat them with the marinade, cover, and refrigerate overnight.
2. Preheat the oven to 400 degrees F. Remove the fish from the fridge and scrape off the marinade. Coat a cast iron skillet with avocado oil, and heat at medium-high. Add the fish, and brown, about 2 minutes per side.
3. Transfer the fillets to the oven and bake until flaky, about 10 minutes.

*Adapted from* Younger *by Sara Gottfried, MD*

# Braised Turmeric-Cinnamon Chicken

Divine comfort food. Pro tip: It's all about the two-hour simmer. Don't cut it short. This dish is delicious served over riced cauliflower and steamed spinach.

*Serves 4 to 6*

> 1 whole chicken with skin, chopped into 8 pieces (or substitute chicken thighs)
> Sea salt to taste
> Freshly ground pepper
> Ground cinnamon
> Turmeric
> 2 tablespoons olive oil
> 1 medium to large yellow onion, chopped
> 4 cloves garlic, chopped
> 2 cinnamon sticks
> 1 14-ounce can whole peeled Italian tomatoes (no sugar added)
> 1–2 cups Chicken Bone Broth (see recipe on page 227)
> Fresh mint and parsley to garnish

1. Wash and dry chicken pieces. Season all over with salt, pepper, and a light sprinkling of ground cinnamon and turmeric.
2. Coat a large pot with olive oil and place over medium heat. When oil is heated, sear chicken pieces for 1 minute on each side, until the skin is browned. Remove chicken pieces from pan and set aside.
3. Lower heat to medium-high and add onions. Stir for 1 minute or until soft, then add garlic. Let cook for another minute, until translucent. Add cinnamon sticks, tomatoes, and broth, and season with salt and pepper. Stir and bring to simmer. Add chicken pieces back into the pot, submerging them in the liquid. Simmer for about 2 hours uncovered, shaking the pan from time to time to move the chicken around, until meat is falling off the bone.
4. Garnish with mint and parsley, and serve.

*Adapted from* Younger *by Sara Gottfried, MD*

# Slow-Cooker Chicken

I love the simplicity of this meal in a pot. Just five ingredients, plus water. You could probably use an Instant Pot (mine is still in the cabinet, untouched). To make sure the chicken is cooked all the way through, make sure the internal temperature gets to 165 degrees at some point during the cooking. This is the perfect nourishing soup to eat when you don't feel well.

*Serves 4 to 8*

> 3 large onions, thinly sliced
> 4–8 cups filtered water (enough to cover chicken)
> 1 pastured whole chicken
> 1 onion, chopped
> 1 cup celery, chopped
> 1 cup carrots, chopped
> Optional: 2 cups spiralized zucchini

1. Assemble the sliced onion, water, and chicken in a slow cooker. Cook on high for 4 to 6 hours or on low for 6 to 8 hours. Add water, if necessary, to keep chicken covered. Add celery and carrots for the last hour of cooking. If desired, add spiralized zucchini as an alternative to noodles.
2. After soup is fully cooked, remove chicken and shred. Place some in the bottom of each soup bowl. Ladle broth and veggies over chicken, and serve.

*Adapted from* Brain Body Diet *by Sara Gottfried, MD*

# Nut-Crusted Chicken Fingers

A crowd-pleaser for both kids and adults. The chicken fingers can be placed on top of a salad or served with a sauce (try the recipe for Pesto on page 223, or use chimichurri or your favorite low-carb hot sauce).

*Serves 2 adults or up to 4 children*

> ½ cup ground nuts (macadamia nuts, almonds, or walnuts)
> ¼ cup ground flax
> ¼ cup sesame seeds
> 1 large pastured egg
> 1 8-ounce pastured boneless skinless chicken thigh, cut
>     into strips

1. In a small bowl, combine the ground nuts, flax, and seeds. In a separate bowl, beat the egg. Place the strips of chicken in the egg to marinate for 5 minutes, flipping the strips to coat as needed.
2. Preheat the oven to 350 degrees F. Cover a large baking tray with parchment paper.
3. Once the chicken is coated well in egg, carefully press each strip into the nut mixture, making sure it is well coated on both sides. Then place the coated chicken on the baking tray. Do not crowd the pieces.
4. Bake for about 20 minutes. Remove the chicken from the oven. Turn the chicken pieces and return them to the oven for another 15 to 20 minutes, until fully cooked and golden.

*Adapted from* Brain Body Diet *by Sara Gottfried, MD*

# Beef and Vegetable Stew

This is one of the hearty soups that prevented hunger cravings for me, leading to success the third time I tried a ketogenic diet.

*Serves 6 to 12*

> 4 tablespoons coconut oil (expeller-pressed)
> 8 cloves garlic, minced
> 2 pounds stew meat from grass-fed beef, cut into bite-sized pieces
> 1 large yellow onion, chopped
> 5 carrots, chopped
> 5–7 stalks celery, chopped
> 1 cup butternut squash, cubed
> Optional: 1 cup red wine (preferably organic; note the alcohol will burn off while cooking)
> 6 bay leaves
> 3 sprigs fresh thyme or ½ teaspoon dried
> 1 sprig fresh rosemary or 1 teaspoon dried
> 1 teaspoon smoked paprika
> 2 quarts Beef Bone Broth (see recipe on page 228)
> Sea salt and pepper to taste
> Optional: 1–2 tablespoons almond butter, to thicken

1. In a heavy stockpot, heat the coconut oil over medium-high heat. Add garlic and meat, and cook until the meat is browned, but be careful not to burn the garlic. Add the vegetables and stir until they are mixed in well with the meat (you may need to add more oil). Add the red wine and cook for 5 to 8 minutes to allow the alcohol to cook off, so it doesn't affect ketosis. Add spices. Stir to combine. Add broth.
2. Cover and bring to a boil, then lower heat to simmer for 1 hour. Taste for salt and seasoning. If you want a thicker stew, add the optional almond butter. Provided the veggies are done, the stew is now ready to eat. But if left to cook at a very low heat for 3 to 4 hours, it will be even tastier.

*Adapted from* Younger *by Sara Gottfried, MD*

# VEGETABLES

## Baked Jerusalem Artichokes with Thyme and Lemon

Jerusalem artichokes are full of prebiotic fiber.

*Serves 4 to 6*

1 ½ cups heavy cream or crème fraîche
Juice of 1 lemon
2 garlic cloves, peeled, smashed, and chopped
1 handful of fresh thyme, chopped
½ cup Parmesan, grated
2 ¼ pounds Jerusalem artichokes, peeled and sliced like a pencil
1 slice keto bread, toasted
Extra-virgin olive oil

1. Preheat oven to 425 degrees F. In medium bowl, mix cream, lemon, garlic, half of the thyme, and most of the Parmesan. Add artichokes and stir to combine.
2. Use food processor to pulse toasted keto bread into crumbs. Add remaining thyme and Parmesan to the food processor and combine. Place artichokes in a gratin dish. Sprinkle with the dry topping and drizzle with olive oil. Bake 30 minutes.

## Roasted Eggplant

I love the delicate taste of Japanese eggplant, but you can substitute other varieties, such as the teardrop-shaped American or the rounded European. For a sauce, try this chapter's recipe for Tahini Dressing or Chermoula.

*Serves 2 to 4*

> 4 Japanese eggplants, sliced into rounds on the diagonal, approximately ½ inch thick
> Spray olive oil or coconut oil
> Sea salt and pepper to taste

1. Preheat oven to 350 degrees F. Set eggplant slices on a parchment-lined baking sheet and spray with oil. Roast until tender, about 15 to 20 minutes. Season with salt and pepper, and serve with the sauce of your choice.

## Steamed Artichokes

Don't be intimidated by the work of cooking and eating artichokes. It's a divinely flavorful vegetable to include in the Gottfried Protocol. The options for dipping will add flavor, along with a dose of healthy fat. If you'd like, make your own mayonnaise (see the recipe for Mayonnaise on page 218), or keep a good brand in your refrigerator (see Resources).

*Serves 2 to 4*

> 2–4 medium artichokes
> 2–4 cloves of garlic, to taste
> 1 bay leaf
> Juice of 1 lemon
> 2–4 tablespoons mayonnaise, melted butter, or ghee,
>     for dipping

1. Trim artichokes — cut off top inch and stem, and use kitchen shears to clip the tips of the pointy leaves. Make sure that the bottom of each artichoke is flat; trim as needed.
2. Fill a pot with several inches of cold water, and add garlic, bay leaf, and lemon juice. Place a steamer basket in the pot and add artichokes. Make sure the water doesn't rise above the bottom of the basket, so that the artichokes steam rather than boil. Cover the pot, bring water to a boil, then reduce heat to a simmer. Steam until the leaves can be plucked easily from the artichoke — about 20 to 30 minutes.
3. To eat: Starting at the base of the artichoke, pluck one leaf at a time. Dip it in mayonnaise or another fat, then pull the base of the leaf through your teeth to scrape away the delicious fleshy part. Continue the process, one leaf at a time. When you come to the fuzzy center, which sits on top of a meaty core known as the heart, scrape away the fibrous fuzz to get to the heart. The edible disk that remains is the best part.

# DESSERT

## Keto Pumpkin Custard

This may sound like a holiday dessert, but it's scrumptious at any time of year.

*Serves 4 to 6*

> 15 ounces canned pumpkin puree (or roast your own, as explained on page 196)
> 2 large pastured eggs
> 1 cup heavy cream
> ¼ cup granulated erythritol sweetener
> 1½ teaspoons pumpkin pie spice
> ½ teaspoon salt
> 1 teaspoon vanilla extract
> Optional: 1 teaspoon xanthan gum

1. Preheat oven to 350 degrees F. Place 4 to 6 ramekins (or small shallow bowls) in a large pan with high enough sides to hold a water bath. Fill a kettle with water, and set to boil.
2. In a large mixing bowl, combine pumpkin puree, eggs, cream, sweetener, spice, salt, vanilla, and xanthan gum, if using. Whisk together until smooth.
3. Divide the mixture among ramekins. Place the whole pan of ramekins into the oven, and then carefully fill the pan with hot water until the water reaches halfway up the sides of the ramekins. (Or, if you prefer, you can fill the pan before putting it in the oven.)
4. Bake for 40 minutes or until set (an inserted knife should emerge mostly clean). Carefully remove the ramekins from the water bath (I use kitchen tongs with rubber bands wrapped around the end of each tong, to get a good grip), and allow custard to cool on a wire rack. Store in the refrigerator.

# No-Bake Coconut Love Bites

These are a healthy alternative to fat bombs! I use organic vanilla extract.

*Serves 12 to 20*

> 3 cups unsweetened shredded coconut
> 6 tablespoons coconut oil
> ½ cup xylitol or erythritol sweetener
> 2 teaspoons vanilla extract
> ½ teaspoon Himalayan sea salt
> Optional toppings: shredded coconut, unsweetened cocoa powder, finely chopped nuts, dark chocolate with stevia — melted for piping or drizzling

1. Put all ingredients (except toppings) into a food processor or blender. Combine until the mixture is blended and sticks together. (Note: If you are using a high-powered blender like a Vitamix, do not turn your machine on high as it may melt the batter.) Remove the mixture from the blender or food processor and form into desired shapes. I usually make balls with a melon scooper.
2. Decorate with toppings as desired. I use a plastic bag with a tiny hole cut in the corner to pipe the chocolate, or you can just drizzle it. You can also leave them plain.
3. Leave to firm up at room temperature on a plate or other hard surface.

*Adapted from* Younger *by Sara Gottfried, MD*

# Almond-Coconut Macaroons

A keto update of the Passover favorite.

*Serves 6 to 12*

> 1 cup almond or coconut flour
> 2 cups unsweetened shredded or flaked coconut
> Optional: 1 teaspoon cocoa powder
> 2 large pastured eggs
> ½ teaspoon salt
> ½ teaspoon vanilla extract
> ½ teaspoon cinnamon powder

1. Preheat oven to 300 degrees F.
2. In a large bowl, mix together the almond flour and shredded coconut. Add the cocoa powder, if using. In a separate bowl, beat together the eggs.
3. Pour the eggs into the flour mixture. Add salt, vanilla, and cinnamon.
4. Wet your hands and form little balls of batter. Pat them tightly together. Place the macaroons at least 1 inch apart on a baking tray lined with parchment paper.
5. Bake for about 15 to 20 minutes, or until cookies are golden in color.

*Adapted from* Brain Body Diet *by Sara Gottfried, MD*

# Dark Chocolate–Coconut Pudding

I eat dessert only twice per week, and this recipe truly satisfies.

*Serves 4*

> 2 cups coconut milk (reserve 2 tablespoons for dissolving
> gelatin)
> 1 tablespoon high-quality unflavored powdered gelatin (a form
> of collagen that is soluble only in hot liquid)
> 3–4 ounces dark chocolate (90 percent cocoa solids), chopped
> into small pieces
> ½ teaspoon vanilla extract
> Pinch of sea salt

1. Reserve 2 tablespoons of the coconut milk. Heat the rest on low in a heavy-bottomed pot.
2. In a separate small pan, mix the reserved coconut milk with the gelatin, and stir over low heat for a few minutes until dissolved; set aside. In the heavy-bottomed pan, add the dark chocolate to the coconut milk and whisk constantly until it melts completely and mixture is smooth.
3. Add the gelatin mixture to the chocolate mixture by slowly pouring it in as you whisk. (If you put it in all at once, the mixture will get clumpy.) Turn off the heat and whisk in the vanilla extract.
4. Pour the pudding into bowls or cups, and chill for at least 2 hours, or until set. Garnish with a pinch of sea salt and serve.

*Adapted from* Younger *by Sara Gottfried, MD*

# Chocolate-Avocado "Ice Cream"

For those who love the frozen stuff — this alternative is much more nutritious.

*Serves 2 to 4*

> 1 avocado, halved, pitted, peeled, and chopped
> 1 can (13 ½ ounces) full-fat coconut milk
> ½ cup unsweetened cocoa powder
> ¼–½ cup erythritol sweetener or monk fruit extract
> ½ cup filtered water
> 2 teaspoons vanilla extract
> ½ teaspoon sea salt

1. Place the avocado and coconut milk in a food processor or blender and combine. Add the remaining ingredients and blend for about 2 minutes, until smooth. You may need to stop partway and scrape down the sides. Freeze the "ice cream" using one of these methods:

MACHINE METHOD

2. Place mixture in the container that came with your ice cream machine, and put in the refrigerator for 2 hours, to set up before freezing. Then prepare and freeze according to the manufacturer's instructions.

HAND METHOD

Place mixture in a freezer-safe container and freeze for 1 hour. Over the next 3 to 4 hours, remove the mixture from the freezer every 20 minutes and whisk it slightly, to prevent it from getting too icy. It should thicken after each whisking until it's firm enough to scoop.

3. Prior to serving, let the "ice cream" thaw a little, for 5 to 10 minutes.

*Adapted from* Brain Body Diet *by Sara Gottfried, MD*

# Avocado-Lime Sorbet

Refreshing and light.

*Serves 2 to 4*

> 2 ripe avocados, halved, pitted, peeled, and chopped
> 2 cups unsweetened almond milk (or filtered water, if you
>    prefer a lighter taste and icier texture)
> ¼–½ cup xylitol or erythritol sweetener or monk fruit extract
> 2 tablespoons fresh lime juice
> 1 tablespoon lime zest
> ½ teaspoon sea salt

1. Place the ingredients in a food processor or blender and combine until smooth. Freeze the sorbet using one of these methods:

   MACHINE METHOD
2. Chill the container that came with your ice cream machine, then place the mixture in it. Prepare and freeze according to the manufacturer's instructions.

   HAND METHOD
   Place the mixture in a freezer-safe container and freeze for 1 hour.

3. Over the next 3 to 4 hours, remove the mixture from the freezer every 20 minutes and whisk it slightly, to prevent it from getting too icy. It should thicken after each whisking until it's firm enough to scoop.
4. Best if eaten within 24 hours.

*Adapted from* Brain Body Diet *by Sara Gottfried, MD*

# MEAL PLANS

Omnivore

| | Day 1 | Day 2 | Day 3 | Day 4 | Day 5 | Day 6 | Day 7 |
|---|---|---|---|---|---|---|---|
| **Breakfast** | Iced Coffee Collagen Shake (page 198) | Green Egg Scramble (page 203) | Deep Green Shake (page 202) | Shakshuka (page 208) | Avo Toast (page 204) | Carrot Cake Shake (page 201) | Almond Butter–Cacao Nib Shake (page 198) |
| **Lunch** | Little Gem Salad (page 211), moderate protein (chicken, salmon, low-mercury tuna)* | Slow Cooker Chicken, spaghetti squash (leftover) | Sorrel Soup (page 232), Nut-Crusted Chicken Fingers (leftover) | Crispy Cucumber Salad with Cilantro-Tahini Dressing (page 214) | Baked Jerusalem Artichokes with Thyme and Lemon (page 248), smoked salmon | Thai Coconut-Chicken Soup (leftover) | Chopped Greens and Marcona Salad (page 212), Gazpacho (page 231) |
| **Dinner** | Slow Cooker Chicken (page 245), spaghetti squash, artichoke | Avgolemono Soup (page 226), green salad, Nut-Crusted Chicken Fingers (page 246) | "Taco" Salad (page 216) | Beef and Vegetable Stew (page 247), green salad | Thai Coconut-Chicken Soup (Tom Kha Gai) (page 234) | Salmon with Almond Crust (see variation, page 242), Halibut with Almond Crust, riced cauliflower | Egg-Avocado Bake (page 209), avocado, green salad |

* Reminder: I recommend 10–20 percent of calories from carbohydrates, 20 percent of calories from protein, and the remaining 60–70 percent from fat.

## Pescatarian

| | Day 1 | Day 2 | Day 3 | Day 4 | Day 5 | Day 6 | Day 7 |
|---|---|---|---|---|---|---|---|
| **Breakfast** | Dark Chocolate–Sea Salt Shake (page 200) | Keto granola, nut milk | Shakshuka (page 208) | Almond Butter–Cacao Nib Shake (page 198) | Golden Milk Shake (page 200) | Green Egg Scramble (page 203) | Avo Toast (page 204) |
| **Lunch** | Little Gem Salad (page 211), moderate protein (chicken, salmon, low-mercury tuna) | Shirataki noodles, Pesto (page 223) | Kale and Caesar Salad with Raw "Parmesan" (page 221), Grilled Salmon Steaks (leftover) | Tahini-Sesame Noodles (leftover) | Torn Greens with Ranch Dressing (page 218), smoked salmon | Basic Green Salad (page 210), Roasted Eggplant (page 249), Fish Bone Broth (page 229) | Crispy Cucumber Salad with Cilantro-Tahini Dressing (page 214) |
| **Dinner** | Frittata with Spinach, Eggplant, and Pine Nuts (page 207) | Grilled Salmon Steaks with Lemon-Herb Mojo (page 241) | Tahini-Sesame Noodles (page 237) | Salmon and Avocado Bowl with Miso Dressing (page 240) | Black Cod with Miso (page 243), riced cauliflower, medium green salad | Roasted fish, Chermoula (page 223), leftover vegetables | Halibut with Almond Crust (page 242) |

## Vegetarian

| | Day 1 | Day 2 | Day 3 | Day 4 | Day 5 | Day 6 | Day 7 |
|---|---|---|---|---|---|---|---|
| **Breakfast** | Carrot Cake Shake (page 201) | Keto granola, nut milk | Dragon Fruit Shake (page 199) | Green Egg Scramble (page 203) | Basic Gottfried Protocol Shake for Ketosis (page 194) | Avo Toast (page 204) | Shakshuka (page 208) |
| **Lunch** | Little Gem Salad (page 211), 2 poached eggs | Tahini-Sesame Noodles (page 237) | Frittata (leftover) | Torn Greens with Ranch Dressing (page 218) | Kimchi, Shirataki, and Bok Choy Bowl (page 238) | Seaweed Salad (page 220) | Sorrel Soup (page 232) |
| **Dinner** | Tea Leaf Salad (page 213) | Frittata with Spinach, Eggplant, and Pine Nuts (page 207) | Tofu Masala Soup (page 235) | Gazpacho (page 231) | Egg-Avocado Bake (page 209) | Vegetable "Fettuccine" Alfredo (page 239) | Baked Jerusalem Artichokes with Thyme and Lemon (page 248) |

## Vegan

| | Day 1 | Day 2 | Day 3 | Day 4 | Day 5 | Day 6 | Day 7 |
|---|---|---|---|---|---|---|---|
| Breakfast | Iced Coffee Collagen Shake (page 198) | Keto granola, nut milk | Deep Green Shake (page 202) | Almond Butter–Cacao Nib Shake (page 198) | Basic Gottfried Protocol Shake for Ketosis (page 194) | Carrot Cake Shake (page 201) | Golden Milk Shake (page 200) |
| Lunch | Little Gem Salad (page 211) | Tahini-Sesame Noodles (page 237) | Avo Toast (page 204) | Crispy Cucumber Salad with Cilantro-Tahini Dressing (page 214) | Seaweed Salad (page 220) | Sorrel Soup (page 232) | French Onion Soup (page 233) |
| Dinner | Cauliflower Ceviche (page 222) | Tofu Masala Soup (page 235) | Gazpacho (page 257) | Vegetable "Fettuccine" Alfredo (page 239) | Baked Jerusalem Artichokes with Thyme and Lemon (page 248) | Kimchi, Shirataki, and Bok Choy Bowl (page 238) | Roasted Eggplant (page 249) |

# RESOURCES

## APPS

- Zero and MyCircadianClock for intermittent fasting.
- Lifesum (use the keto setting) or MyFitnessPal for macronutrients.
- Calm, Headspace, Ten Percent Happier for meditation.
- Peloton and Glo-Yoga for yoga and meditation.

## DEVICES

You don't need all of these. Most important are the Renpho scale and Keto-mojo.

- Renpho scale — a Bluetooth body-composition scale. I want you to lose fat and preserve muscle mass, and this $30 scale will help. It may not be the most accurate, but the trends over time can be helpful.
- Blood ketone monitor — Keto-mojo and Precision Extra.
- Glucose monitor — Precision Xtra Blood Glucose and Ketone Monitoring System and Contour next EZ. Both require that

you prick your finger for a drop of blood, and the meters plus supplies are available at drugstores and online. I prefer the Precision because it allows you to also check your blood ketones, and both glucose and ketones may be helpful to monitor while on the Gottfried Protocol.

- Continuous glucose monitor: Abbott FreeStyle Libre, DexCom.
- Oura ring — for sleep, exercise, and recovery tracking.
- Apolloneuro.com — a wearable wellness device for stress relief.
- Urine ketone strips — I don't use them, but some people like them.

## TESTS TO CONSIDER

These are tests that I commonly order in my precision medicine practice. You might want to discuss them with your physician or physical trainer.

- Body composition.
- Resting metabolic rate.
- Exercise performance, such as VO2 max.
- Continuous glucose monitoring.
- Laboratory testing.

You can also order your own clinical laboratory tests from Wellnessfx.com and Yourlabwork.com.

Here are additional genomic and biomarker tests that I recommend. For the following tests, I recommend that you review results with a functional medicine clinician, even for the direct-to-consumer testing:

**Genomic testing**

**3x4 Genetics** https://www.3x4genetics.com/

**DNA Life** https://www.dnalife.healthcare/

**Genomind** https://www.genomind.com/

**Genova Diagnostics** https://www.gdx.net/

> **DetoxiGenomic Profile:** www.gdx.net/core/sample
> -reports/DetoxiGenomics-Sample-Report.pdf

> **EstroGenomic Profile:** www.gdx.net/core/support-guides/
> Estro-Genomic-

## Gut, microbiota, and microbiome testing

**Gastrointestinal Microbial Assay Plus (GI-MAP)** by
Diagnostic Solutions Lab, https://www.diagnosticsolutionslab
.com/tests/gi-map

**GI360 Microbiome** Profile by Doctor's Data, https://www
.doctorsdata.com/gi-360/

**GI Effects** by Genova, https://www.gdx.net/product/gi-effects
-comprehensive-stool-test

**GutBio** by Onegevity, https://www.onegevity.com/
products/gutbio

**Organic Acids Test** by Great Plains Laboratory, https://www.
greatplainslaboratory.com/organic-acids-test

## Hormone testing

Dried urine test for comprehensive hormones (DUTCH) by
Precision Analytical https://dutchtest.com

**Complete Hormones** test by Genova: www.gdx.net/product/
complete-hormones-test-urine

**Essential Estrogens** by Genova: www.gdx.net/product/essential
-estrogens-hormone-test-urine

## Micronutrient testing

**NutrEval** by Genova. This test documents micronutrient
deficiencies and heavy metals in the blood and urine and

provides information about personalized supplementation need for antioxidants, amino acids, B vitamins, digestive support, essential fatty acids, and minerals. www.gdx.net/product/nutreval-fmv-nutritional-test-blood-urine

**Metabolomix** by Genova. This test provides many of the same features as the NutrEval but can be performed at home with blood spot and urine specimens. https://www.gdx.net/product/metabolomix+nutritional-test-urine

**Micronutrient Test** by Spectracell. This test is preferred by my mentor, Mark Houston MD, for assessing cellular deficiencies and insufficiencies relevant to cardiovascular disease. https://www.spectracell.com/micronutrient-test-panel

# KITCHENWARE

**Cast iron skillets.** These are my go-to pans for cooking. A little iron will scrape off and get in your food, so make sure you do not have excess iron in your body before using.

**Enameled cast iron.** I bought my first Le Creuset enameled cast iron Dutch oven from a used cooking store in San Francisco when I was an intern in medicine back in 1994. My collection continues to serve most every need, particularly for making bone broths and soups that cook for hours to days.

**GreenPan.** Ceramic nonstick, toxin-free cookware featuring the Thermolon coating, free of toxins like perfluorooctanoic acid (PFOA), per- and polyfluroalkyl substances (PFAS), lead, and cadmium. Dishwasher- and metal utensil–safe.

**ScanPan.** Environmentally progressive nonstick pans made in Denmark and free of PFOA and PFOS, the toxins in Teflon, yet these pans provide a durable nonstick surface. The Classic Fry Pan is the most versatile pan in my collection (9.5 inch/24 cm).

**Vitamix.** I buy a new Vitamix about once every three years, when my ice cubes no longer blend to smooth. It is unparalleled in blending performance. Certified reconditioned blenders are available at their website.

# FOOD

Success on the Gottfried Protocol requires creativity and innovation in finding swaps for refined carbs like pasta, rice, cereal, and bread. Here are my favorite swaps:

- Bread becomes keto bread, which is denser (see Recipes for Tahini Bread on page 206 and Coffee Cake on page 205, or check out the brand recommended on the next list).
- Cereal becomes keto granola (see brands that follow).
- Crackers become flackers or vegetable crudités (celery sticks, sliced zucchini, radishes, sliced carrots, sliced squash).
- Pasta becomes spiralized zucchini, squash, turnip, or other vegetables (see Recipes), or shirataki or konjac (see brands that follow).
- Rice becomes riced cauliflower or shirataki rice.
- Brownies become keto brownies.
- Cookies become keto cookies.
- Potato chips become oven-baked pork rinds — they can also be ground up as a swap for breadcrumbs or panko.

**Keto bread:** Make your own, or buy Base Culture Original Keto Bread (Baseculture.com), which has 4 net carbs per slice (8 grams of carbs, 4 grams of fiber, 6 grams of fat, 4 grams of protein). Made from water, eggs, almond butter, flaxseed, arrowroot flour, psyllium husk, almond flour, and apple cider vinegar, it's grain-free, gluten-free, preservative-free, and dairy-free. I keep several loaves in my freezer for making grilled cheese or vegan cucumber sandwiches, or I add nut or seed butter for a quick snack.

**Brownies:** I love the High Key Brownie Baking Mix in Blondie Original (1 net carb) or Chocolate Chip Fudge (2 net carbs). Be attentive to serving size!

**Cereal:** For cold cereal, choose a keto granola with less than 5 net carbs per serving. (Be sure to weigh out the serving, as they should be small yet are nutrient dense.) My favorite brands include Low Karb Cacao (3 net carbs) made with almonds, pecans, and coconut, and Cinnamon Pecan (2 net carbs). Other brands include Julian Bakery Keto Granola in Peanut Butter Cinnamon (3 net carbs) or High Key Cinnamon Almond (2 net carbs). For warm cereal, I like High Key Keto Instant Hot Cereal in Cocoa Almond or Strawberries and Cream (both 2 net carbs).

**Chocolate:** I like the Chocolate Zero keto bark and dark chocolate peanut-butter cups. I keep Lily's sugar-free chocolate chips on hand and mix them with 1 tablespoon of nut butter.

**Flax crackers:** My favorite crackers are made from flax and are available at flackers.com. (I also use Forti-Flax premium ground flaxseed by Barlean's in my shakes and my keto Coffee Cake recipe.)

**Vegetables:** I keep hardy vegetables in the refrigerator (broccoli, kale, bok choy, celery, collard greens, eggplant, and lettuce, especially romaine). Some I keep in the freezer (broccoli, riced cauliflower, and greens such as kale, spinach, and collards). For travel, I use Poshi packets of asparagus and French beans, packed in vinegar and extra-virgin olive oil, and ready to eat. I also travel with Urban Remedy sour cream and chive kale chips, and a low-carb Rainbow salad, both vegan (Urbanremedy.com).

**Salmon:** I travel with packets of smoked salmon (less than 1 carb) or salmon jerky (0 carbs) from Alaska Smokehouse (wwgormet.com).

**Tuna:** I like Safe Catch Elite wild tuna, sustainably wild-caught and tested for mercury. I like the chili-lime flavor and travel with packets of these.

**Snacks:** If you like a crunchy, salty snack, consider High Key Goat Cheese snack bags. I travel with these too. I have a casein intolerance but can tolerate these in rotation (every four days or so). Another choice is Epic Oven Baked Pork Rinds. These come in a variety of flavors — I like chili-lime or Himalayan salt. I've tried vegan options, but they are too high in carbs for me. I travel with grass-fed beef jerky and beef sticks, including the New Primal Sea Salt Beef Thins.

## SUPPLEMENTS

**Alpha-lipoic acid:** I like Stabilized R-Lipoic Acid Supreme by Designs for Health.

**Balanced omegas:** I like EFA-Sirt Supreme from Biotics Research because it has a balanced blend of the essential fatty acids EPA, DHA, and GLA, together with mixed tocopherols, specially formulated to be high in gamma ($\gamma$)-tocopherol. You can also make your own mix of EPA and DHA (I take 4 grams per day), and add either GLA (I like Metagenics and take 2–3 grams per day) or separately from evening primrose oil (6 percent GLA), borage oil (24 percent GLA), or black currant oil (17 percent GLA).

**Electrolytes:** I use Designs for Health Electropure (0 grams carbs), ½ teaspoon in 8 to 12 ounces of filtered water.

**Medium-chain triglyceride chews:** When you are first starting on keto, these chews can help get you into ketosis more quickly and improve focus and energy. Many of my patients find them helpful in the afternoon to prevent alcohol cravings. I use them when traveling. I recommend Designs for Health KTO-C8

MCT Oil Chews with 500 mg caprylic acid, in strawberry/watermelon flavor.

**Specialized pro-resolving mediators:** In the United States, there are two companies that manufacture SPMs with high-quality standards: Designs for Health and Metagenics. I recommend either brand. Follow the instructions on the bottle for dosage.

# ACKNOWLEDGMENTS

There are innumerable people to thank, and I am sure I will miss many. Deep gratitude to my patients and cases for this book; they keep me humble and curious about why fat loss is so challenging as we age.

I'm grateful to the friends and colleagues who generously helped me clarify and organize my thinking: Drs. Rachel Abrams, Erin Amato, Anthony Bazzan, Melissa Blake, Sheldon Cohen, Anu French, Victoria Hall, Mark Houston, Laura Konigsberg, Daniel Monti, Myles Spar, and Will Van Derveer. Special thanks for the outstanding editing by Pamela Walter. While writing this book, I was moved by a timely lecture on the role of axiology, or the study of values, and how values motivate behavior change. The talk was given by Keith Kurlander, cofounder (along with Dr. Will Van Derveer) of the Integrative Psychiatry Institute. Thank you, Keith, for connecting the dots between values and behavior change!

My extraordinary agent, Celeste Fine, continues to lead me forward with tremendous grace, insight, and wit.

Once I embarked on a book about women, food, and hormones, I couldn't have done it without my extraordinary editorial, design, social media, and launch teams: Deb Brody, Topher Donahue, Maya

Dusenbery, Nathalie Hadi, Sharon Kastoriano, Eve Minkler, Sarah Pelz, Emma Peters, Shara Alexander, and Kevin Plottner. Special thanks to our digital and tech team: Kenny Gregg and Barry Napier.

I am grateful to the woman who helps create calm in our home: Leslie Murphy.

Thank you to my loving family, including my brilliant daughters, who keep me honest about feminism, intersectionality, and body-positive language. I'm grateful to my dog daughter, Juneau, for reminding me that it's time to play. Thank you to my beloved parents, Albert and Mary.

Heartfelt thanks to Johanna Ilfeld, PhD, one of my best friends and fitness partner, who read draft after draft with abiding affection, irreverence, and wisdom; and David Gottfried, my husband, life partner, and greatest love.

# NOTES

## INTRODUCTION:
## THE LANGUAGE OF HORMONES

1. Diabetes Prevention Program Research Group, "10-Year Follow-Up of Diabetes Incidence and Weight Loss in the Diabetes Prevention Program Outcomes Study," *The Lancet* 374, no. 9702 (2009): 1677–86; R. B. Goldberg et al., "Targeting the Consequences of the Metabolic Syndrome in the Diabetes Prevention Program," *Arteriosclerosis, Thrombosis, and Vascular Biology* 32, no. 9 (2012): 2077–90; Diabetes Prevention Program Research Group, "Long-Term Effects of Lifestyle Intervention or Metformin on Diabetes Development and Microvascular Complications over 15-year Follow-Up: The Diabetes Prevention Program Outcomes Study," *The Lancet Diabetes & Endocrinology* 3, no. 11 (2015): 866–75.

2. P. Garrido et al., "Proposal for the Creation of a National Strategy for Precision Medicine in Cancer: A Position Statement of SEOM, SEAP, and SEFH," *Clinical and Translational Oncology* 20, no. 4 (2018): 443–47; G. Gonzalez-Hernandez et al., "Advances in Text Mining and Visualization for Precision Medicine," *Biocomputing* 23 (2018): 559–65; C. A. L. Wicklund et al., "Clinical Genetic Counselors: An Asset in the Era of Precision Medicine," *American Journal of Medical Genetics, Part C: Seminars in Medical Genetics* 178, no. 1 (2018): 63–67; "Precision Medicine," *National Institutes of Health*, https://olao.od.nih.gov/content/precision-medicine, accessed September 18, 2020.

3. "The Truth Is Out There, Somewhere," *Lancet* 396, no. 10247 (2020): 291.

4. T. N. Seyfried et al., "Role of Glucose and Ketone Bodies in the Metabolic Control of Experimental Brain Cancer," *British Journal of Cancer* 89, no. 7 (2003): 1375–82; L. M. Rodrigues et al., "The Action of β-hydroxybutyrate on the Growth,

Metabolism, and Global Histone H3 Acetylation of Spontaneous Mouse Mammary Tumours: Evidence of a β-hydroxybutyrate Paradox," *Cancer & Metabolism* 5, no. 1 (2017): 4–17; C. Bartmann et al., "Beta-hydroxybutyrate (3-OHB) Can Influence the Energetic Phenotype of Breast Cancer Cells but Does Not Impact Their Proliferation and the Response to Chemotherapy or Radiation," *Cancer & Metabolism* 6, no. 1 (2018): 8; M. Chen et al., "An Aberrant SREBP-Dependent Lipogenic Program Promotes Metastatic Prostate Cancer," *Nature Genetics* 50, no. 2 (2018): 206–18; G. Kolata, "High-Fat Diet May Fuel Spread of Prostate Cancer," *The New York Times,* January 16, 2018, https://www.nytimes.com/2018/01/16/health/fat-diet-prostate-cancer.html, accessed August 15, 2018; J. Sremanakova et al., "A Systematic Review of the Use of Ketogenic Diets in Adult Patients with Cancer," *Journal of Human Nutrition and Dietetics* 3, no. 6 (2018): 793–802.

5. G. Bonuccelli et al., "Ketones and Lactate 'Fuel' Tumor Growth and Metastasis: Evidence That Epithelial Cancer Cells Use Oxidative Mitochondrial Metabolism," *Cell Cycle* 9, no. 17 (2010): 3506–14; U. E. Martinez-Outschoorn et al., "Ketones and Lactate Increase Cancer Cell 'Stemness,' Driving Recurrence, Metastasis, and Poor Clinical Outcome in Breast Cancer: Achieving Personalized Medicine Via Metabolo-Genomics," *Cell Cycle* 10, no. 8 (2011): 1271–86.

6. S. E. Swithers, "Artificial Sweeteners Produce the Counterintuitive Effect of Inducing Metabolic Derangements," *Trends in Endocrinology & Metabolism* 24, no. 9 (2013): 431–41.

7. J. S. Volek et al., "Cardiovascular and Hormonal Aspects of Very-Low-Carbohydrate Ketogenic Diets," *Obesity Research* 12, no. S11 (2004): 115S–123S; J. S. Volek et al., "Comparison of Energy-Restricted Very-Low-Carbohydrate and Low-Fat Diets on Weight Loss and Body Composition in Overweight Men and Women," *Nutrition & Metabolism* 1, no. 13 (2004): 1–13; H. M. Dashti et al., "Long-Term Effects of Ketogenic Diet in Obese Subjects," *Molecular and Cellular Biochemistry* 286, no. 1–2 (2006): 1–9; G. Ruaño, "Physiogenomic Analysis of Weight Loss Induced by Dietary Carbohydrate Restriction," *Nutrition & Metabolism* 3, no. 1 (2006): 3–20; K. Durkalec-Michalski et al., "Effect of a Four-Week Ketogenic Diet on Exercise Metabolism in CrossFit-Trained Athletes," *Journal of the International Society of Sports Nutrition* 16, no. 1 (2019): 16.

8. The higher fat intake in women was in the setting of relatively high carbohydrate intake (51 percent of total calories per day), not a ketogenic diet. S. L. Mumford et al., "Dietary Fat Intake and Reproductive Hormone Concentrations and Ovulation in Regularly Menstruating Women," *The American Journal of Clinical Nutrition* 103, no. 3 (2016): 868–77.

9. J. M. Wilson et al., "The Effects of Ketogenic Dieting on Body Composition, Strength, Power, and Hormonal Profiles in Resistance Training Males," *The Journal of Strength and Conditioning Research* (2017); A. R. Kuchkuntla et al., "Ketogenic Diet: An Endocrinologist Perspective," *Current Nutrition Reports* 8, no. 4 (2019): 402–10.

10. When it comes to healthy gut microbiota, what matters is the type, quality, quan-

tity, and origin of the food. Gut bugs utilize nutrients in the food you consume for basic biological functions (such as regulating the immune system) and then create metabolic outputs that impact your physiology — including energy balance, glucose signaling, inflammation, and fat loss. One of the most important nutrients for a healthy microbiome is microbiota-accessible carbohydrates, such as prebiotic fiber. The key to success on the Gottfried Protocol is to get sufficient quantities of these specific carbs and to feed the good bugs.

F. Bäckhed et al., "The Gut Microbiota as an Environmental Factor That Regulates Fat Storage," *Proceedings of the National Academy of Sciences of the United States of America* 101, no. 44 (2004): 15718–723; M. Rescigno, "Intestinal Microbiota and Its Effects on the Immune System," *Cellular Microbiology* 16, no. 7 (2014): 1004–13; L. Geurts et al., "Gut Microbiota Controls Adipose Tissue Expansion, Gut Barrier, and Glucose Metabolism: Novel Insights into Molecular Targets and Interventions Using Prebiotics," *Beneficial Microbes* 5, no. 1 (2014): 3–17; B. O. Schroeder et al., "Signals from the Gut Microbiota to Distant Organs in Physiology and Disease," *Nature Medicine* 22, no. 10 (2016): 1079–89; K. Makki, "The Impact of Dietary Fiber on Gut Microbiota in Host Health and Disease," *Cell Host & Microbe* 23, no. 6 (2018): 705–15.

11. R. de Cabo et al., "Effects of Intermittent Fasting on Health, Aging, and Disease," *New England Journal of Medicine* 381, no. 26 (2019): 2541–51.

12. Note that intermittent fasting increases neurogenesis, the ongoing growth and development of new nerve cells (that is, neurons, which contribute to functions like learning, emotional regulation, and memory). B. Malinowski, "Intermittent Fasting in Cardiovascular Disorders — An Overview," *Nutrients* 11, no. 3 (2019): 673; A. L. Mindikoglu, Intermittent Fasting from Dawn to Sunset for 30 Consecutive Days Is Associated with Anticancer Proteomic Signature and Upregulates Key Regulatory Proteins of Glucose and Lipid Metabolism, Circadian Clock, DNA Repair, Cytoskeleton Remodeling, Immune System, and Cognitive Function in Healthy Subjects," *Journal of Proteomics* 217 (2020): 103645; S. H. Baik et al., "Intermittent Fasting Increases Adult Hippocampal Neurogenesis," *Brain and Behavior* 10, no. 1 (2020): e01444.

13. Intermittent fasting decreases total cholesterol, LDL-cholesterol (known colloquially as the "bad" type), and serum triglycerides. It reduces fat accumulation in the liver and fat tissues. G. M. Tinsley et al., "Effects of Intermittent Fasting on Body Composition and Clinical Health Markers in Humans," *Nutrition Reviews* 73, no. 10 (2015): 661–74; A. Bener et al., "Effect of Ramadan Fasting on Glycemic Control and Other Essential Variables in Diabetic Patients," *Annals of African Medicine* 17, no. 4 (2018): 196; A. R. Rahbar et al., "Effects of Intermittent Fasting During Ramadan on Insulin-like Growth Factor-1, Interleukin 2, and Lipid Profile in Healthy Muslims," *International Journal of Preventive Medicine* 10, no. 7 (2019): 1–6; S. Ebrahimi et al., "Ramadan Fasting Improves Liver Function and Total Cholesterol in Patients with Nonalcoholic Fatty Liver Disease," *International Journal for Vitamin and Nutrition Research* (2019).

14. B. H. Goodpaster et al., "Metabolic Flexibility in Health and Disease," *Cell Metabolism* 25, no. 5 (2017): 1027–36

15. https://www.cdc.gov/media/releases/2020/s0917-adult-obesity-increasing.html, accessed September 29, 2020.

16. N. Stefan et al., "Causes, Characteristics, and Consequences of Metabolically Unhealthy Normal Weight in Humans," *Cellular Metabolism* 26, no. 2 (2017): 292–300; N. Stefan et al., "Obesity and Impaired Metabolic Health in Patients with COVID-19," *Nature Reviews Endocrinology* (2020): 1–2.

17. S. Y. Tartof, et al. "Obesity and Mortality Among Patients Diagnosed With CO-VID-19: Results from an Integrated Health Care Organization," *Annals of Internal Medicine* (2020): M20-3742; W. Dietz et al., "Obesity and Its Implications for CO-VID-19 Mortality," *Obesity (Silver Spring)* 28, no. 6 (2020): 1005; A. Simonnet et al., "High Prevalence of Obesity in Severe Acute Respiratory Syndrome Coronavirus-2 (SARS-CoV-2) Requiring Invasive Mechanical Ventilation," *Obesity (Silver Spring)* 28, no. 7 (2020): 1195–99; Erratum in *Obesity (Silver Spring)* 28, no. 10 (2020): 1994; B. M. Popkin et al., "Individuals with Obesity and COVID-19: A Global Perspective on the Epidemiology and Biological Relationships," *Obesity Reviews* (2020) Aug 26:10.1111/obr.13128.

18. L. Gupta et al., "Ketogenic Diet in Endocrine Disorders: Current Perspectives," *Journal of Postgraduate Medicine* 63, no. 4 (2017): 242–51.

## 1. THE TRUTH ABOUT
## WOMEN, HORMONES, AND WEIGHT

1. My outstanding acupuncturist, Emily Hooker, provides the following insights about traditional Chinese medicine (TCM) and hormones in women: "While traditional Chinese medicine texts do not explicitly acknowledge perimenopause, female life cycles are thought to occur in seven-year phases, with 42 being the age that the shao yang (gallbladder, associated with liver) begins to decline. That said, they also assert that a woman's hair turns white in that phase, which seems dated and potentially lifestyle-based. Just as you write that cortisol dysregulation is at the root of many patterns, this can be said of LQS, and yes, sighing is definitely an indication that there's a LQS component.

Over time, LQS has the potential to cause a host of other imbalances, often beginning with spleen qi deficiency. This could be at the root of any metabolic issue, though seldom as a singular diagnosis. Either way, that has no bearing on the accuracy of your assessment of Melissa, who certainly presents with LQS. Incidentally, I am seeing a 44-year-old female patient at the moment with a nearly identical picture. Her cortisol levels are high, progesterone and testosterone are low, thyroid is underactive, and she also gained about 20 pounds within the past year. Her TCM diagnosis is liver qi stagnation with spleen qi and yang deficiency causing dampness." To learn more from Emily, go to emilyhookeracupuncture.com.

2. P. K. Whelton et al., "ACC/AHA/AAPA/ABC/ACPM/AGS/APhA/ASH/ASPC/ NMA/PCNA Guideline for the Prevention, Detection, Evaluation, and Manage-

ment of High Blood Pressure in Adults: Executive Summary: A Report of the American College of Cardiology/American Heart Association Task Force on Clinical Practice Guidelines," *Hypertension* 71, no. 6 (2018): 1269–1324.

3. B. V. Howard et al., "Insulin Resistance and Weight Gain in Postmenopausal Women of Diverse Ethnic Groups," *International Journal Obesity and Related Metabolism Disorder* 28, no. 8 (2004): 1039–47; O. T. Hardy et al., "What Causes the Insulin Resistance Underlying Obesity?" *Current Opinion Endocrinology, Diabetes, and Obesity* 19, no. 2 (2012): 81–87; H. U. Moon et al., "The Association of Adiponectin and Visceral Fat with Insulin Resistance and β-Cell Dysfunction," *Journal of Korean Medical Science* 34, no. 1 (2018): e7; J. Fatima et al., "Association of Sonographically Assessed Visceral and Subcutaneous Abdominal Fat with Insulin Resistance in Prediabetes," *Journal of the Association Physicians of India* 67, no. 4 (2019): 68–70.

4. J. Rezzonico et al., "Introducing the Thyroid Gland as Another Victim of the Insulin Resistance Syndrome," *Thyroid* 18, no. 4 (2008): 461–64; C. Anil et al., "Metformin Decreases Thyroid Volume and Nodule Size in Subjects with Insulin Resistance: A Preliminary Study," *Medical Principles and Practice* 25, no. 3 (2016): 233–36; C. Sallorenzo et al., "Prevalence of Pancreatic Autoantibodies in Non-Diabetic Patients with Autoimmune Thyroid Disease and Its Relation to Insulin Secretion and Glucose Tolerance," *Archives of Endocrinology and Metabolism* 61, no. 4 (2017): 361–66; P. Zhu et al., "Thyroid-Stimulating Hormone Levels Are Positively Associated with Insulin Resistance," *Medical Science Monitor* 24, no. 1 (2018): 342–47; U. Mousa et al., "Fat Distribution and Metabolic Profile in Subjects with Hashimoto's Thyroiditis," *Acta Endocrinologica* 14, no. 1 (2018): 105–12; X. Zhang et al., "Effect of Insulin on Thyroid Cell Proliferation, Tumor Cell Migration, and Potentially Related Mechanisms," *Endocrine Research* 44, nos. 1–2 (2019): 55–70; X. He et al., "Role of Metformin in the Treatment of Patients with Thyroid Nodules and Insulin Resistance: A Systematic Review and Meta-Analysis," *Thyroid* 29, no. 3 (2019): 359–67.

5. A. Verma et al., "Hypothyroidism and Obesity? Cause or Effect," *Saudi Medical Journal* 29, no. 8 (2008): 1135–38; R. Song et al., "The Impact of Obesity on Thyroid Autoimmunity and Dysfunction: A Systematic Review and Meta-Analysis," *Frontiers in Immunology* 10, no. 1 (2019): 2349.

6. R. C. Kessler et al., "Lifetime and 12-Month Prevalence of DSM-III-R Psychiatric Disorders in the United States," *Archives of General Psychiatry* 51, no. 1 (1994): 8–19; R. C. Kessler et al., "Posttraumatic Stress Disorder in the National Comorbidity Survey," *Archives of General Psychiatry* 52, no. 12 (1995): 1048–60; M. Altemus et al., "Sex Differences in Anxiety and Depression Clinical Perspectives," *Frontiers in Neuroendocrinology* 35, no. 3 (2014): 320–30.

7. L. Fan et al., "Non-linear Relationship Between Sleep Duration and Metabolic Syndrome: A Population-Based Study," *Medicine (Baltimore)* 99, no. 2 (2020): e18753.

8. B. L. Fredrickson et al., "Objectification Theory: Toward Understanding Women's

Lived Experiences and Mental Health Risks," *Psychology of Women Quarterly* 21, no. 2 (1997): 173–206; C. Rollero et al., "Self-Objectification and Personal Values: An Exploratory Study," *Frontiers in Psychology* 8, no. 1 (2017): 1055; R. Kahalon et al., "Experimental Studies on State Self-Objectification: A Review and an Integrative Process Model," *Frontiers in Psychology* 9, no. 1 (2018): 1268.

9. L. M. Schaefer et al., "Self-Objectification and Disordered Eating: A Meta-Analysis," *The International Journal of Eating Disorders* 51, no. 6 (2018): 483–502.

10. L. Cheng, "The Commercialization of Female Bodies in Consumer Society," *Journal of Humanity* 9, no. 1 (2015): 123–25.

11. M. P. J. Vanderpump, "The Epidemiology of Thyroid Disease," *British Medical Bulletin* 99, no. 1 (2011): 39–51; R. Hoermann et al., "Recent Advances in Thyroid Hormone Regulation: Toward a New Paradigm for Optimal Diagnosis and Treatment," *Frontiers in Endocrinology* 8, no. 1 (2017): 364; A. G. Juby et al., "Clinical Challenges in Thyroid Disease: Time for a New Approach?" *Maturitas* 87, no. 1 (2016): 72–78.

12. D. M. Roesch, "Effects of Selective Estrogen Receptor Agonists on Food Intake and Body Weight Gain in Rats," *Physiology & Behavior* 87, no. 1 (2006): 39–44; A. L. Hirschberg, "Sex Hormones, Appetite, and Eating Behaviour in Women," *Maturitas* 71, no. 3 (2012): 248–56; L. Asarian et al. "Sex Differences in the Physiology of Eating," *American Journal of Physiology-Regulatory, Integrative, and Comparative Physiology* 305, no. 11 (2013): R1215–67.

13. G. D. Miller et al., "Basal Growth Hormone Concentration Increased Following a Weight Loss Focused Dietary Intervention in Older Overweight and Obese Women," *The Journal of Nutrition, Health, & Aging* 16, no. 2 (2012): 169–74.

14. M. Devaki et al., "Chronic Stress-Induced Oxidative Damage and Hyperlipidemia Are Accompanied by Atherosclerotic Development in Rats," *Stress* 16, no. 2 (2013): 233–43; S. N. Kales et al., "Firefighters and On-Duty Deaths from Coronary Heart Disease: A Case Control Study," *Environmental Health* 2, no. 1 (2003): 14; M. Kumari et al., "Chronic Stress Accelerates Atherosclerosis in the Apolipoprotein E Deficient Mouse," *Stress* 6, no. 4 (2003): 297–99; H. E. Webb et al., "Stress Reactivity to Repeated Low-Level Challenges: A Pilot Study," *Applied Psychophysiology Biofeedback* 36, no. 4 (2011): 243–50.

15. P. M. Peeke et al., "Hypercortisolism and Obesity," *Annals of New York Academy of Science* 771, no. 1 (1995): 665–76; S. Paredes et al., "Cortisol: The Villain in Metabolic Syndrome?" *Revista da Associacao Medica Brasileria (1992)* 60, no. 1 (2014): 84–92; J. Q. Purnell et al., "Enhanced Cortisol Production Rates, Free Cortisol, and 11beta-HSD-1 Expression Correlate with Visceral Fat and Insulin Resistance in Men: Effect of Weight Loss," *American Journal of Physiology Endocrinology and Metabolism* 296, no. 2 (2000): E351–57; A. Tchernof et al., "Pathophysiology of Human Visceral Obesity: An Update," *Physiological Reviews* 93, no. 1 (2013): 359–404.

16. M. J. McAllister et al., "Exogenous Carbohydrate Reduces Cortisol Response

from Combined Mental and Physical Stress," *International Journal of Sports Medicine* 37, no. 14 (2016): 1159–65.

17. C. J. Ley et al., "Sex- and Menopause-Associated Changes in Body-Fat Distribution," *The American Journal of Clinical Nutrition* 55, no. 5 (1992): 950–54.

18. L. M. Brown et al., "Central Effects of Estradiol in the Regulation of Food Intake, Body Weight, and Adiposity," *The Journal of Steroid Biochemistry and Molecular Biology* 122, nos. 1–3 (2010): 65–73.

19. Ley et al., "Sex- and Menopause-Associated Changes."

20. Q. Cao et al., "Waist-Hip Ratio as a Predictor of Myocardial Infarction Risk: A Systematic Review and Meta-Analysis," *Medicine* 97, no. 30 (2018); V. A. Benites-Zapata VA et al., "High Waist-to-Hip Ratio Levels Are Associated with Insulin Resistance Markers in Normal-Weight Women," *Diabetes Metabolic Syndrome* 13, no. 1 (2019): 636–42.

21. B. Tramunt et al., "Sex Differences in Metabolic Regulation and Diabetes Susceptibility," *Diabetologia* 63, no. 3 (2020): 453–61.

22. V. Regitz-Zagrosek et al., "Gender Aspects of the Role of the Metabolic Syndrome as a Risk Factor for Cardiovascular Disease," *Gender Medicine* 4 (2007): S162–77; E. Gerdts et al., "Sex Differences in Cardiometabolic Disorders," *Nature Medicine* 25, no. 11 (2019): 1657–66.

23. S. V. Ahn et al., "Sex Difference in the Effect of the Fasting Serum Glucose Level on the Risk of Coronary Heart Disease," *Journal of Cardiology* 71, no. 2 (2018): 149–54.

24. G. A. Greendale et al., "Changes in Body Composition and Weight During the Menopause Transition," *JCI Insight* 4, no. 5 (2019).

25. A. M. Goss et al., "Longitudinal Associations of the Endocrine Environment on Fat Partitioning in Postmenopausal Women," *Obesity (Silver Spring)* 20, no. 5 (2012): 939–44; S. Ballestri et al., "NAFLD as a Sexual Dimorphic Disease: Role of Gender and Reproductive Status in the Development and Progression of Nonalcoholic Fatty Liver Disease and Inherent Cardiovascular Risk," *Advances in Therapy* 34, no. 6 (2017): 1291–326.

26. J. R. Guthrie et al., "Weight Gain and the Menopause: A 5-Year Prospective Study," *Climacteric: The Journal of the International Menopause Society* 2, no. 3 (1999): 205–11.

27. S. L. Crawford et al., "A Longitudinal Study of Weight and the Menopause Transition: Results from the Massachusetts Women's Health Study," *Menopause (New York, N.Y.)* 7, no. 2 (2000): 96–104.

28. S. C. Ho et al., "Menopausal Transition and Changes of Body Composition: A Prospective Study in Chinese Perimenopausal Women," *International Journal of Obesity (2005)* 34, no. 8 (2010): 1265–74.

29. F. Fery et al., "Hormonal and Metabolic Changes Induced by an Isocaloric Isoproteinic Ketogenic Diet in Healthy Subjects," *Diabète & Métabolisme* 8, no. 4 (1982): 299–305; E. Kose et al., "Changes of Thyroid Hormonal Status in Patients

Receiving Ketogenic Diet Due to Intractable Epilepsy," *Journal of Pediatric Endocrinology & Metabolism* 30, no. 4 (2017): 411–16; Y. J. Lee et al., "Longitudinal Change in Thyroid Hormone Levels in Children with Epilepsy on a Ketogenic Diet: Prevalence and Risk Factors," *Journal of Epilepsy Research* 7, no. 2 (2017): 99–105.

30. For a complete list of hypothyroid symptoms, see pages 30–31 and Chapter 9 of my book *The Hormone Cure: Reclaim Balance, Sleep, Sex Drive, and Vitality Naturally with the Gottfried Protocol* (New York: Simon and Schuster, 2013).

31. J. Sirven et al., "The Ketogenic Diet for Intractable Epilepsy in Adults: Preliminary Results," *Epilepsia* 40, no. 12 (1999): 1721–26.

32. R. M. Kwan et al., "Effects of a Low Carbohydrate Isoenergetic Diet on Sleep Behavior and Pulmonary Functions in Healthy Female Adult Humans," *Journal of Nutrition* 116, no. 12 (1986): 2393–402.

33. A. A. Prather et al., "Poor Sleep Quality Potentiates Stress-Induced Cytokine Reactivity in Postmenopausal Women with High Visceral Abdominal Adiposity," *Brain, Behavior, Immunity* 35, no. 1 (2014): 155–62; S. K. Sweatt et al., "Sleep Quality Is Differentially Related to Adiposity in Adults," *Psychoneuroendocrinology* 98, no. 1 (2018): 46–51.

34. In this research study of the ketogenic diet in rats, investigators used microcomputed tomography and histomorphometry analyses on the distal femur. They found trabecular bone volume, serum IGF-I, and the bone formation marker P1NP were lower in male rats fed a low-carb, high-fat diet. A. Zengin et al., "Low-Carbohydrate, High-Fat Diets Have Sex-Specific Effects on Bone Health in Rats," *European Journal of Nutrition* 55, no. 7 (2016): 2307–20.

35. G. K. Schwalfenberg, "The Alkaline Diet: Is There Evidence That an Alkaline pH Diet Benefits Health?" *Journal of Environmental and Public Health* 2012, no. 1 (2012): 727630.

36. B. E. Millen et al., "The 2015 Dietary Guidelines Advisory Committee Scientific Report: Development and Major Conclusions," *Advances in Nutrition* 7, no. 3 (2016): 438–44; Q. Qian, "Dietary Influence on Body Fluid Acid-Base and Volume Balance: The Deleterious 'Norm' Furthers and Cloaks Subclinical Pathophysiology," *Nutrients* 10, no. 6 (2018): 778.

37. Acid and alkaline refer to pH: acids have a low pH of less than 7, and alkaline has a high pH of more than 7. The pH of blood is 7.4, but foods can leave an acidic or alkaline ash. L. Frassetto et al., "Diet, Evolution and Aging—The Pathophysiologic Effects of the Post-Agricultural Inversion of the Potassium-to-Sodium and Base-to-Chloride Ratios in the Human Diet," *European Journal of Nutrition* 40, no. 5 (2001): 200–213; M. Konner et al., "Paleolithic Nutrition: Twenty-Five Years Later," *Nutrition in Clinical Practice* 25, no. 6 (2010): 594–602. J. R. Buendia et al., "Longitudinal Effects of Dietary Sodium and Potassium on Blood Pressure in Adolescent Girls," *JAMA Pediatrics* 169, no. 6 (2015): 560–68; A. Sebastian et al., "Postulating the Major Environmental Condition Resulting in the Expression of Essential Hypertension and Its Associated Cardiovascular Diseases: Dietary Im-

prudence in Daily Selection of Foods in Respect of Their Potassium and Sodium Content Resulting in Oxidative Stress-Induced Dysfunction of the Vascular Endothelium, Vascular Smooth Muscle, and Perivascular Tissues," *Medical Hypotheses* 119, no. 1 (2018): 110–19.

38. S. T. Reddy et al., "Effect of Low-Carbohydrate High-Protein Diets on Acid-Base Balance, Stone-Forming Propensity, and Calcium Metabolism," *American Journal of Kidney Diseases* 40, no. 2 (2002): 265–74; E. H. Kossoff et al., "Dietary Therapies for Epilepsy," *Biomed Journal* 36, no. 1 (2013): 2–8.

39. L. Frassetto et al., "Potassium Bicarbonate Reduces Urinary Nitrogen Excretion in Postmenopausal Women," *The Journal of Clinical Endocrinology & Metabolism* 82, no. 1 (1997): 254–59; L. Frassetto et al., "Long-term Persistence of the Urine Calcium-Lowering Effect of Potassium Bicarbonate in Postmenopausal Women," *The Journal of Clinical Endocrinology & Metabolism* 90, no. 2 (2005): 831–34; J. A. Wass et al., "Growth Hormone and Memory," *The Journal of Endocrinology* 207, no. 2 (2010): 125–26; G. K. Schwalfenberg, "The Alkaline Diet: Is There Evidence That an Alkaline pH Diet Benefits Health?" *Journal of Environmental and Public Health* 2012, no. 1 (2012): 727630.

40. R. Solianik et al., "Two-Day Fasting Evokes Stress, but Does Not Affect Mood, Brain Activity, Cognitive, Psychomotor, and Motor Performance in Overweight Women," *Behavioural Brain Research* 338, no. 1 (2018): 166–72.

41. R. Solianik et al., "Effect of 48H Fasting on Autonomic Function, Brain Activity, Cognition, and Mood in Amateur Weight Lifters," *Biomed Research International* 2016, no. 1 (2016): 1503956.

## 2. HOW GROWTH HORMONE KEEPS YOU LEAN

1. J. D. Veldhuis et al., "Somatotropic and Gonadotropic Axes Linkages in Infancy, Childhood, and the Puberty-Adult Transition," *Endocrine Reviews* 27, no. 2 (2006): 101–40; J. D. Veldhuis, "Aging and Hormones of the Hypothalamo-Pituitary Axis: Gonadotropic Axis in Men and Somatotropic Axes in Men and Women," *Ageing Research Reviews* 7, no. 3 (2008): 189–208.

2. E. Corpas et al., "Human Growth Hormone and Human Aging," *Endocrine Reviews* 14, no. 1 (1993): 20–39; A. Bartke, "Growth Hormone and Aging: Updated Review," *The World Journal of Men's Health* 37, no.1 (2019): 19–30.

3. S. Perrini et al., "Metabolic Implications of Growth Hormone Therapy," *Journal of Endocrinological Investigation — Supplements* 31, no. 9 (2008): 79–84; S. Perrini et al., "Abnormalities of Insulin-like Growth Factor-I Signaling and Impaired Cell Proliferation in Osteoblasts from Subjects with Osteoporosis," *Endocrinology* 149, no. 3 (2007): 1302–13; K. R. Short et al., "Enhancement of Muscle Mitochondrial Function by Growth Hormone," *The Journal of Clinical Endocrinology & Metabolism* 93, no. 2 (2008): 597–604; N. Møller et al., "Effects of Growth Hormone on Glucose, Lipid, and Protein Metabolism in Human Subjects," *Endocrine Reviews* 30, no. 2 (2009): 152–77.

4. L. I. Arwert et al., "The Relation Between Insulin-Like Growth Factor I Levels

and Cognition in Healthy Elderly: A Meta-Analysis." *Growth hormone & IGF Research* 15, no. 6 (2005): 416–422.

5. U. J. Lewis, "Growth Hormone: What Is It and What Does It Do?" *Trends in Endocrinology & Metabolism* 3, no. 4 (1992): 117–21; M. B. Ranke et al., "Growth Hormone—Past, Present, and Future." *Nature Reviews Endocrinology* 14, no. 5 (2018): 285–300.

6. F. Mourkioti et al., "IGF-1, Inflammation, and Stem Cells: Interactions During Muscle REGEneration," *Trends in Immunology* 26, no. 10 (2005): 535–42; C. P. Velloso, "Regulation of Muscle Mass by Growth Hormone and IGF-I," *British Journal of Pharmacology* 154, no. 1 (2008): 557–68, M. E. Molitch et al., "Evaluation and Treatment of Adult Growth Hormone Deficiency: An Endocrine Society Clinical Practice Guideline," *The Journal of Clinical Endocrinology & Metabolism* 96, no. 6 (2011): 1587–609.

7. A. L. Cardoso et al., "Towards Frailty Biomarkers: Candidates from Genes and Pathways Regulated in Aging and Age-Related Diseases," *Ageing Research Reviews* 47, no. 1 (2018): 214–77.

8. G. Vab den Berg et al., "An Amplitude-Specific Divergence in the Pulsatile Mode of Growth Hormone (GH) Secretion Underlies the Gender Difference in Mean Growth Hormone Concentrations in Men and Premenopausal Women," *Journal of Clinical Endocrinology and Metabolism* 81, no. 7 (1996): 2460–67; J. O. Jørgensen et al., "Sex Steroids and the Growth Hormone/Insulin-like Growth Factor-I Axis in Adults," *Hormone Research in Paediatrics* 64, Suppl. 2 (2005): 37–40.

9. G. Norstedt et al., "Secretory Rhythm of Growth Hormone Regulates Sexual Differentiation of Mouse Liver," *Cell* 36, no. 4 (1984): 805–12.

10. F. Roelfsema et al., "Growth-Hormone Dynamics in Healthy Adults Are Related to Age and Sex, and Strongly Dependent on Body Mass Index," *Neuroendocrinology* 103, nos. 3–4 (2016): 335–44; J. P. Span et al., "Gender Difference in Insulin-Like Growth Factor I Response to Growth Hormone (GH) Treatment in Growth Hormone–Deficient Adults: Role of Sex Hormone Replacement," *Journal of Clinical Endocrinology Metabolism* 85, no. 3 (2000): 1121–25.

11. A. Eliakim et al., "Effect of Gender on the Growth Hormone-IGF-I Response to Anaerobic Exercise in Young Adults," *Journal of Strength and Conditioning Research* 28, no. 12, (2014): 3411–15.

12. M. Russell-Aulet et al., "Aging-Related Growth Hormone Decrease Is a Selective Hypothalamic Growth Hormone–Releasing Hormone Pulse Amplitude Mediated Phenomenon," *The Journals of Gerontology, Series A: Biological Sciences and Medical Sciences* 56, no. 2 (2001): M124–29.

13. N. Vahl et al., "Abdominal Adiposity and Physical Fitness Are Major Determinants of the Age-Associated Decline in Stimulated Growth Hormone Secretion in Healthy Adults," *The Journal of Clinical Endocrinology & Metabolism* 81, no. 6 (1996): 2209–215.

14. M. Misra et al., "Lower Growth Hormone and Higher Cortisol Are Associated

with Greater Visceral Adiposity, Intramyocellular Lipids, and Insulin Resistance in Overweight Girls," *American Journal of Physiology-Endocrinology and Metabolism* 295, no. 2 (2008): E385–92.

15. I. Fukuda et al., "Serum Adiponectin Levels in Adult Growth Hormone Deficiency and Acromegaly," *Growth Hormone & IGF Research* 14, no. 6 (2004): 449–54; R. Stawerska et al., "Relationship Between IGF-I Concentration and Metabolic Profile in Children with Growth Hormone Deficiency: The Influence of Children's Nutritional State as Well as the Ghrelin, Leptin, Adiponectin, and Resistin Serum Concentrations," *International Journal of Endocrinology* 2017 (2017); E. Witkowska-Sędek et al., "The Associations Between the Growth Hormone/Insulin-like Growth Factor-1 Axis, Adiponectin, Resistin, and Metabolic Profile in Children with Growth Hormone Deficiency Before and During Growth Hormone Treatment," *Acta Biochimica Polonica* 65, no. 2 (2018): 333–40.

16. Z. P. Li et al., "Study of the Correlation Between Growth Hormone Deficiency and Serum Leptin, Adiponectin, and Visfatin Levels in Adults," *Genetics and Molecular Research: GMR* 13, no. 2 (2014): 4050–56.

17. J. D. Veldhuis et al., "Distinctive Inhibitory Mechanisms of Age and Relative Visceral Adiposity on Growth Hormone Secretion in Pre-and Postmenopausal Women Studied Under a Hypogonadal Clamp," *The Journal of Clinical Endocrinology & Metabolism* 90, no. 11 (2005): 6006–13.

18. Li et al., "Study of the Correlation Between Growth."

19. The complete list of hormones that are involved in regulating growth hormone and/or IGF-1 include estrogen, cortisol (that is, adrenocorticotropic hormone), thyroid (specifically, the control hormone for thyroid production, thyrotropin releasing hormone), luteinizing hormone, follicle-stimulating hormone, human chorionic gonadotropin (the hormone of pregnancy), insulin, other growth factors (for example, platelet-derived growth factor [PDGF], epidermal growth factor [EGF], and fibroblast growth factors [FGFs]), combined with age, sex, diet, nutrition, and other lifestyle factors. A. Kasprzak et al., "Insulin-like Growth Factor (IGF) Axis in Cancerogenesis." *Mutation Research/Reviews in Mutation Research* 772, no. 1 (2017): 78–104.

20. I recommend a full hormone panel to my patients, including thyroid stimulating hormone or TSH, free T3, free T4, reverse T3, thyroid peroxidase antibodies, and anti-thyroglobulin antibodies. Additional thyroid tests may be indicated, checking on symptoms. See Resources for recommended labs that perform this type of testing without a doctor's orders, but please work with a collaborative health-care practitioner to interpret results.

21. E. Giovannucci et al., "Nutritional Predictors of Insulin-like Growth Factor I and Their Relationships to Cancer in Men," *Cancer Epidemiology, Biomarkers, & Prevention* 12, no. 2 (2003): 84–89.

22. S. C. Larsson et al., "Association of Diet with Serum Insulin-like Growth Factor I in Middle-Aged and Elderly Men," *The American Journal of Clinical Nutrition* 81, no. 5 (2005): 1163–67.

23. M. Holmes et al., "Dietary Correlates of Plasma Insulin-like Growth Factor I and Insulin-like Growth Factor Binding Protein 3 Concentrations," *Cancer Epidemiology, Biomarkers, & Prevention* 11, no. 9 (2002): 852–61.

24. S. M. Phillips et al., "Dietary Protein for Athletes: From Requirements to Optimum Adaptation," *Journal of Sports Sciences* 29, Suppl. 1 (2011): S29–38; M. Huecker et al., "Protein Supplementation in Sport: Source, Timing, and Intended Benefits," *Current Nutrition Reports* 8, no. 4 (2019): 382–396.

25. K. Zhu et al., "The Effects of a Two-Year Randomized, Controlled Trial of Whey Protein Supplementation on Bone Structure, IGF-1, and Urinary Calcium Excretion in Older Postmenopausal Women," *Journal of Bone and Mineral Research* 26, no. 9 (2011): 2298–306.

26. J. M. Bauer et al., "Effects of a Vitamin D and Leucine-Enriched Whey Protein Nutritional Supplement on Measures of Sarcopenia in Older Adults, The PROVIDE Study: A Randomized, Double-Blind, Placebo-Controlled Trial," *Journal of the American Medical Directors Association* 16, no. 9 (2015): 740–47; M. Rondanelli et al., "Whey Protein, Amino Acids, and Vitamin D Supplementation with Physical Activity Increases Fat-Free Mass and Strength, Functionality, and Quality of Life and Decreases Inflammation in Sarcopenic Elderly," *The American Journal of Clinical Nutrition* 103, no. 3 (2016): 830–40; S. Verlaan et al., "Sufficient Levels of 25-Hydroxyvitamin D and Protein Intake Required to Increase Muscle Mass in Sarcopenic Older Adults — The PROVIDE Study," *Clinical Nutrition* 37, no. 2 (2018): 551–57.

27. E. Castillero et al., "Comparison of the Effects of the n-3 Polyunsaturated Fatty Acid Eicosapentaenoic and Fenofibrate on the Inhibitory Effect of Arthritis on IGF1," *Journal of Endocrinology* 210, no. 3 (2011): 361–68.

28. In the omega-3 pathway, several problems can upregulate an enzyme called delta-5-desaturase, which leads to production of more arachidonic acid, an inflammatory fat. These problems include essential hypertension, cardiovascular disease, insulin resistance, obesity, and metabolic syndrome.

    C. Russo et al., "Increased Membrane Ratios of Metabolite to Precursor Fatty Acid in Essential Hypertension," *Hypertension* 29, no. 4 (1997): 1058–63; B. Vessby, "Dietary Fat, Fatty Acid Composition in Plasma and the Metabolic Syndrome," *Current Opinion in Lipidology* 14, no. 1 (2003): 15–19; T. Domei et al., "Ratio of Serum n-3 to n-6 Polyunsaturated Fatty Acids and the Incidence of Major Adverse Cardiac Events in Patients Undergoing Percutaneous Coronary Intervention," *Circulation Journal* 76, (2012): 423–29; K. Inoue et al., "Low Serum Eicosapentaenoic Acid/Arachidonic Acid Ratio in Male Subjects with Visceral Obesity," *Nutrition & Metabolism* 10, no. 1 (2013): 25; E. Warensjö et al., "Fatty Acid Composition and Estimated Desaturase Activities Are Associated with Obesity and Lifestyle Variables in Men and Women," *Nutrition, Metabolism, and Cardiovascular Diseases* 16, no. 2 (2006): 128–36.

29. B. Yang et al., "Ratio of n-3/n-6 PUFAs and Risk of Breast Cancer: A Meta-Analy-

sis of 274135 Adult Females from 11 Independent Prospective Studies," *BMC Cancer* 14, no. 1 (2014): 105.

30. T. J. Merimee et al., "Diet-Induced Alterations of Growth Hormone Secretion in Man," *Journal of Clinical Endocrinology Metabolism* 42, no. 5 (1976): 931–37; K. Y. Ho et al., "Fasting Enhances Growth Hormone Secretion and Amplifies the Complex Rhythms of Growth Hormone Secretion in Man," *Journal of Clinical Investigation* 81, no. 4 (1988): 968–75; H. Nørrelund et al., "Modulation of Basal Glucose Metabolism and Insulin Sensitivity by Growth Hormone and Free Fatty Acids During Short-Term Fasting," *European Journal Endocrinology* 150, no. 6 (2004): 779–87; H. Nørrelund, "The Metabolic Role of Growth Hormone in Humans with Particular Reference to Fasting," *Growth Hormone & IGF Research* 15, no. 2 (2005): 95–122.

31. H. E. Bergan et al., "Nutritional State Modulates Growth Hormone–Stimulated Lipolysis," *General and Comparative Endocrinology* 217–218 (2015): 1–9.

32. B. D. Horne et al., "Relation of Routine, Periodic Fasting to Risk of Diabetes Mellitus, and Coronary Artery Disease in Patients Undergoing Coronary Angiography," *American Journal of Cardiology* 109, no. 11 (2012): 1558–62.

33. R. Gatti et al., "IGF-I/IGFBP System: Metabolism Outline and Physical Exercise." *Journal of Endocrinological Investigation* 35, no. 7 (2012): 699–707.

34. J. Leppäluoto et al., "Heat Exposure Elevates Plasma Immunoreactive Growth Hormone–Releasing Hormone Levels in Man," *The Journal of Clinical Endocrinology & Metabolism* 65, no. 5 (1987): 1035–38; J. Sirviö et al., "Adenohypophyseal Hormone Levels During Hyperthermia," *Endocrinologie* 25, no. 1 (1987): 21–23; K. Kukkonen-Harjula et al., "How the Sauna Affects the Endocrine System," *Annals of Clinical Research* 20, no. 4 (1988): 262–66; K. Kukkonen-Harjula et al., "Haemodynamic and Hormonal Responses to Heat Exposure in a Finnish Sauna Bath," *European Journal of Applied Physiology and Occupational Physiology* 58, no. 5 (1989): 543–50; D. Jezová et al., "Sex Differences in Endocrine Response to Hyperthermia in Sauna," *Acta Physiologica Scandinavica* 150, no. 3 (1994): 293–98.

35. R. Lammintausta et al., "Change in Hormones Reflecting Sympathetic Activity in the Finnish Sauna," *Annals of Clinical Research* 8, no. 4 (1976): 266–71.

36. M. Välimäki et al., "Effect of Ethanol on Serum Concentrations of Somatomedin C and the Growth hormone (GH) Secretion Stimulated by the Releasing Hormone (GHRH)," *Alcohol and Alcoholism* 1 (1987): 557–59; L. Dees et al., "Effects of Ethanol During the Onset of Female Puberty," *Neuroendocrinology* 51, no. 1 (1990): 64–69; M. Välimäki et al., "The Pulsatile Secretion of Gonadotropins and Growth Hormone, and the Biological Activity of Luteinizing Hormone in Men Acutely Intoxicated with Ethanol," *Alcoholism: Clinical and Experimental Research* 14, no. 6 (1990): 928–31; N. Rachdaoui et al., "Pathophysiology of the Effects of Alcohol Abuse on the Endocrine System," *Alcohol Research: Current Reviews* 38, no. 2 (2017): 255–76.

37. A. De Spiegeleer et al., "Pharmacological Interventions to Improve Muscle Mass,

Muscle Strength, and Physical Performance in Older People: An Umbrella Review of Systematic Reviews and Meta-Analyses," *Drugs & Aging* 35, no. 8 (2018): 719–34.

38. A. R. Martineau et al., "Vitamin D Supplementation to Prevent Acute Respiratory Tract Infections: Systematic Review and Meta-Analysis of Individual Participant Data," *British Medical Journal* (2017): 356: i6583.

39. M. R. Blackman et al., "Growth Hormone and Sex Steroid Administration in Healthy Aged Women and Men: A Randomized Controlled Trial," *Journal of the American Medical Association* 288, no. 18 (2002): 2282–92; H. Liu et al., "Systematic Review: The Safety and Efficacy of Growth Hormone in the Healthy Elderly," *Annals of Internal Medicine* 146, no. 2 (2007): 104–15.

40. S. M. Orme et al., "Mortality and Cancer Incidence in Acromegaly: A Retrospective Cohort Study," *The Journal of Clinical Endocrinology & Metabolism* 83, no. 8 (1998): 2730–34; W. E. Sonntag et al., "Adult-Onset Growth Hormone and Insulin-Like Growth Factor I Deficiency Reduces Neoplastic Disease, Modifies Age-Related Pathology, and Increases Life Span," *Endocrinology* 146, no. 7 (2005): 2920–32; A. J. Swerdlow et al., "Cancer Risks in Patients Treated with Growth Hormone in Childhood: The SAGhE European Cohort Study," *The Journal of Clinical Endocrinology & Metabolism* 102, no. 5 (2017): 1661–72.

41. J. Berlanga-Acosta et al., "Synthetic Growth Hormone–Releasing Peptides (GHRPs): A Historical Appraisal of the Evidences Supporting Their Cytoprotective Effects," *Clinical Medicine Insights: Cardiology* 11, no. 1 (2017); J. T. Sigalos et al., "Growth Hormone Secretagogue Treatment in Hypogonadal Men Raises Serum Insulin-Like Growth Factor-1 Levels," *American Journal Men's Health* 11, no. 6 (2017): 1752–57; J. T. Sigalos et al., "The Safety and Efficacy of Growth Hormone Secretagogues," *Sexual Medicine Reviews* 6, no. 1 (2018).

42. B. C. Nindl et al., "Insulin-like Growth Factor I as a Biomarker of Health, Fitness, and Training Status," *Medicine and Science in Sports and Exercise* 42, no. 1 (2010): 39–49.

## 3. TESTOSTERONE: IT'S NOT JUST FOR MEN

1. C. Longcope, "Adrenal and Gonadal Androgen Secretion in Normal Females," *Clinics in Endocrinology and Metabolism* 15, no. 2 (1986): 213–28.

2. S. L. Davison et al., "Androgen Levels in Adult Females: Changes with Age, Menopause, and Oophorectomy," *The Journal of Clinical Endocrinology & Metabolism* 90, no. 7 (2005): 3847–53.

3. To test your testosterone, I recommend asking your health-care practitioner for a blood test that includes total and free testosterone (that is, the amount that is biologically available to exert effects on your cells). See if they will also measure bioavailable testosterone. You can test DHEA, testosterone, and its downstream hormones in your urine. Next best is to test yourself at the labs that I use for my patients, including WellnessFx.com and DUTCHtest.com. More are mentioned in Resources.

4. Davison et al., "Androgen Levels in Adult Females."

5. N. Orentreich et al., "Age Changes and Sex Differences in Serum Dehydroepian-drosterone Sulfate Concentrations Throughout Adulthood," *Journal of Clinical Endocrinology Metabolism* 59, no. 3 (1984): 551–55.

6. Davison et al., "Androgen Levels in Adult Females"; R. Haring et al., "Age-Specific Reference Ranges for Serum Testosterone and Androstenedione Concentrations in Women Measured by Liquid Chromatography-Tandem Mass Spectrometry," *Journal of Clinical Endocrinology Metabolism* 97, no. 2 (2012): 408–15.

7. C. M. Coenen et al., "Changes in Androgens During Treatment with Four Low-Dose Contraceptives," *Contraception* 53, no. 3 (1996): 171–76; Y. Zimmerman et al., "The Effect of Combined Oral Contraception on Testosterone Levels in Healthy Women: A Systematic Review and Meta-Analysis," *Human Reproductive Update* 20, no. 1 (2014): 76–105; N. Zethraeus et al., "Combined Oral Contraceptives and Sexual Function in Women — A Double-Blind, Randomized, Placebo-Controlled Trial," *Journal of Clinical Endocrinology Metabolism* 101, no. 11 (2016): 4046–53; S. Both et al., "Hormonal Contraception and Female Sexuality: Position Statements from the European Society of Sexual Medicine (ESSM)," *Journal of Sexual Medicine* 16, no. 11 (2019): 1681–95.

8. Statins deplete CoQ10, selenium, selenoproteins, omega 3FA, tocopherols and tocotrienols, K2, other fat soluble vitamins, Heme A, carnitine, free T3, creatine, copper, and zinc. Practitioners, see IFM Tool Kit at IFM.org for further information. P. H. Langsjoen et al., "The Clinical Use of HMG CoA-Reductase Inhibitors and the Associated Depletion of Coenzyme Q10: A Review of Animal and Human Publications," *Biofactors* 18, nos. 1–4 (2003): 101–11; C. R. Harper et al., "Evidence-Based Management of Statin Myopathy," *Current Atherosclerosis Reports* 12, no. 5 (2010): 322–30; H. Qu et al., "Effects of Coenzyme Q10 on Statin-Induced Myopathy: An Updated Meta-Analysis of Randomized Controlled Trials," *Journal of the American Heart Association* 7, no. 19 (2018): e009835.

9. J. Y. Shin et al., "Are Cholesterol and Depression Inversely Related? A Meta-Analysis of the Association Between Two Cardiac Risk Factors," *Annals of Behavioral Medicine* 36, no. 1 (2008): 33–43; G. Corona et al., "The Effect of Statin Therapy on Testosterone Levels in Subjects Consulting for Erectile Dysfunction," *Journal of Sexual Medicine* 7, no. 4, part 1 (2010): 1547–56; E. J. Giltay et al., "Salivary Testosterone: Associations with Depression, Anxiety Disorders, and Antidepressant Use in a Large Cohort Study," *Journal of Psychosomatic Research* 72, no. 3 (2012): 205–13; G. Roberto et al., "Statin-Associated Gynecomastia: Evidence Coming from the Italian Spontaneous ADR Reporting Database and Literature," *European Journal of Clinical Pharmacology* 68, no. 6 (2012): 1007–11; C. M. Schooling et al., "The Effect of Statins on Testosterone in Men and Women: A Systematic Review And Meta-Analysis of Randomized Controlled Trials," *BMC Medicine* 11, no. 1 (2013): 57.

10. L. Mernone et al., "Psychobiological Factors of Sexual Functioning in Aging Women — Findings from the Women 40+ Healthy Aging Study," *Frontiers in Psychology* 10, no. 1 (2019): 546.

11. S. R. Davis et al., "Circulating Androgen Levels and Self-Reported Sexual Function in Women," *Journal of the American Medical Association* 294, no. 1 (2005): 91–96.

12. R. Basson et al., "Role of Androgens in Women's Sexual Dysfunction," *Menopause* 17, no. 5 (2010): 962–71; S. Wåhlin-Jacobsen et al., "Is There a Correlation Between Androgens and Sexual Desire in Women?" *Journal of Sexual Medicine* 12, no. 2 (2015): 358–73.

13. Mernone et al., "Psychobiological Factors of Sexual Functioning."

14. S. R. Davis et al., "Global Consensus Position Statement on the Use of Testosterone Therapy for Women," *The Journal of Clinical Endocrinology and Metabolism* 104, no. 10 (2019): 4660–66.

15. C. Bentley et al., "Dehydroepiandrosterone: A Potential Therapeutic Agent in the Treatment and Rehabilitation of the Traumatically Injured Patient," *Burns & Trauma* 7, no. 26 (2019).

16. H. E. Nagels et al., "Androgens (dehydroepiandrosterone or testosterone) for Women Undergoing Assisted Reproduction," *Cochrane Database of Systemic Reviews* 11, no. 1 (2015).

17. G. P. Williams, "The Role of Oestrogen in the Pathogenesis of Obesity, Type 2 Diabetes, Breast Cancer, and Prostate Disease," *European Journal of Cancer Prevention* 19, no. 4 (2010): 256–71; J. McHenry et al., "Sex Differences in Anxiety and Depression: Role of Testosterone," *Front Neuroendocrinology* 35, no. 1 (2014): 42–57; F. Saad, "The Emancipation of Testosterone from Niche Hormone to Multi-System Player," *Asian Journal of Andrology* 17, no. 1 (2015): 58–60; L. Y. Hui et al., "Association Between MKP-1, BDNF, and Gonadal Hormones with Depression on Perimenopausal Women," *Journal of Women's Health* 25, no. 1 (2016): 71–77; S. Rovira-Llopis et al., "Low Testosterone Levels Are Related to Oxidative Stress, Mitochondrial Dysfunction, and Altered Subclinical Atherosclerotic Markers in Type 2 Diabetic Male Patients," *Free Radical Biology & Medicine* 108, no. 1 (2017): 155–62; H. O. Santos, "Ketogenic Diet and Testosterone Increase: Is the Increased Cholesterol Intake Responsible? To What Extent and Under What Circumstances Can There Be Benefits?" *Hormones (Athens)* 16, no. 3 (2017): 150–60.

18. X. Zhang et al., "Postmenopausal Plasma Sex Hormone Levels and Breast Cancer Risk over 20 Years of Follow-Up," *Breast Cancer Research and Treatment* 137, no. 3 (2013): 883–92; R. T. Fortner et al., "Premenopausal Endogenous Steroid Hormones and Breast Cancer Risk: Results from the Nurses' Health Study II," *Breast Cancer Research* 15, no. 2 (2013): R19; Endogenous Hormones and Breast Cancer Collaborative Group et al., "Sex Hormones and Risk of Breast Cancer in Premenopausal Women: A Collaborative Reanalysis of Individual Participant Data from Seven Prospective Studies," *The Lancet Oncology* 14, no. 10 (2013): 1009–19; R. Kaaks et al., "Premenopausal Serum Sex Hormone Levels in Relation to Breast Cancer Risk, Overall and by Hormone Receptor Status — Results from the EPIC Cohort," *International Journal of Cancer* 134, no. 8 (2014): 1947–57; R. Glaser et al., "Testosterone and Breast Cancer Prevention," *Maturitas* 82, no. 3 (2015): 291–

95; K. A. Bertrand et al., "Circulating Hormones and Mammographic Density in Premenopausal Women," *Hormones & Cancer* 9, no. 2 (2018): 117–27.

19. J. L. Shifren et al., "Transdermal Testosterone Treatment in Women with Impaired Sexual Function After Oophorectomy," *New England Journal of Medicine* 343, no. 10 (2000): 682–88; R. Goldstat et al., "Transdermal Testosterone Therapy Improves Well-Being, Mood, and Sexual Function in Premenopausal Women," *Menopause* 10, no. 5 (2003): 390–98; E. J. Hermans et al., "Exogenous Testosterone Attenuates the Integrated Central Stress Response in Healthy Young Women," *Psychoneuroendocrinology* 32, nos. 8–10 (2007): 1052–61; K. K. Miller et al., "Low-Dose Transdermal Testosterone Augmentation Therapy Improves Depression Severity in Women," *CNS Spectrums* 14, no. 12 (2009): 688–94.

20. B. C. Trainor et al. "Testosterone Promotes Paternal Behaviour in a Monogamous Mammal via Conversion to Oestrogen," *Proceedings of the Royal Society of London, Series B: Biological Sciences* 269, no. 1493 (2002): 823–29.

21. Metabolic problems associated with PCOS include glucose intolerance, metabolic syndrome, and type 2 diabetes. L. J. Moran et al., "Impaired Glucose Tolerance, Type 2 Diabetes, and Metabolic Syndrome in Polycystic Ovary Syndrome: A Systematic Review and Meta-Analysis," *Human Reproduction Update* 16, no. 4 (2010): 347–63; N. S. Kakoly et al., "Ethnicity, Obesity, and the Prevalence of Impaired Glucose Tolerance and Type 2 Diabetes in PCOS: A Systematic Review and Meta-Regression," *Human Reproduction Update* 24, no. 4 (2018): 455–67.

Mental health problems associated with PCOS include anxiety, depression, body dissatisfaction, and lower quality of life. S. Elsenbruch et al., "Quality of Life, Psychosocial Well-Being, and Sexual Satisfaction in Women with Polycystic Ovary Syndrome," *The Journal of Clinical Endocrinology & Metabolism* 88, no. 12 (2003): 5801–7; M. J. Himelein et al., "Depression and Body Image Among Women with Polycystic Ovary Syndrome," *Journal of Health Psychology* 11, no. 4 (2006): 613–25; L. M. Pastore et al., "Depression Symptoms and Body Dissatisfaction Association Among Polycystic Ovary Syndrome Women," *Journal of Psychosomatic Research* 71, no. 4 (2011): 270–76; A. F. Nasiri et al., "The Experience of Women Affected by Polycystic Ovary Syndrome: A Qualitative Study from Iran," *International Journal of Endocrinology and Metabolism* 12, no. 2 (2014); C. Kaczmarek et al., "Health-related Quality of Life in Adolescents and Young Adults with Polycystic Ovary Syndrome: A Systematic Review," *Journal of Pediatric and Adolescent Gynecology* 29, no. 6 (2016): 551–57.

22. L. J. Moran et al., "Sex Hormone Binding Globulin, but Not Testosterone, Is Associated with the Metabolic Syndrome in Overweight and Obese Women with Polycystic Ovary Syndrome," *Journal of Endocrinological Investigation* 36, no. 11 (2013): 1004–10.

23. X. Zhang et al., "The Effect of Low Carbohydrate Diet on Polycystic Ovary Syndrome: A Meta-Analysis of Randomized Controlled Trials," *International Journal of Endocrinology* 2019, no. 4386401 (2019): 1–14.

24. J. C. Mavropoulos et al., "The Effects of a Low-Carbohydrate, Ketogenic Diet on

the Polycystic Ovary Syndrome: A Pilot Study," *Nutrition & Metabolism (Lond)* 2, no. 35 (2005); G. Muscogiuri et al., "Current Insights into Inositol Isoforms, Mediterranean, and Ketogenic Diets for Polycystic Ovary Syndrome: From Bench to Bedside," *Current Pharmaceutical Design* 22, no. 36 (2016): 5554–57; R. K. Stocker et al., "Ketogenic Diet and Its Evidence-Based Therapeutic Implementation in Endocrine Diseases," *Praxis (Bern 1994)* 108, no. 8 (2019): 541–53 (article in German; abstract available in German from the publisher).

25. L. Chen et al., "Sugar-Sweetened Beverage Intake and Serum Testosterone Levels in Adult Males 20–39 Years Old in the United States," *Reproductive Biology Endocrinology* 16, no. 1 (2018).

26. Note that the drink contained 30 grams of glucose and 30 grams of protein. A. Schwartz et al., "Acute Decrease in Serum Testosterone After a Mixed Glucose and Protein Beverage in Obese Peripubertal Boys," *Clinical Endocrinology* 83, no. 3 (2015): 332–38.

27. Note that the drink contained 75 grams of glucose. L. M. Caronia et al., "Abrupt Decrease in Serum Testosterone Levels After an Oral Glucose Load in Men: Implications for Screening for Hypogonadism," *Clinical Endocrinology* 78, no. 2 (2013): 291–96.

28. N. M. Wedick et al., "The Effects of Caffeinated and Decaffeinated Coffee on Sex Hormone–Binding Globulin and Endogenous Sex Hormone Levels: A Randomized Controlled Trial," *Nutrition Journal* 11, no. 1 (2012): 86.

29. K. C. Schliep et al., "Serum Caffeine and Paraxanthine Concentrations and Menstrual Cycle Function: Correlations with Beverage Intakes and Associations with Race, Reproductive Hormones, and Anovulation in the BioCycle Study," *The American Journal of Clinical Nutrition* 104, no. 1 (2016): 155–63.

30. R. L. Ferrini et al., "Caffeine Intake and Endogenous Sex Steroid Levels in Postmenopausal Women: The Rancho Bernardo Study," *American Journal of Epidemiology* 144, no. 7 (1996): 642–44.

31. D. Hang et al., "Coffee Consumption and Plasma Biomarkers of Metabolic and Inflammatory Pathways in US Health Professionals," *The American Journal of Clinical Nutrition* 109, no. 3 (2019): 635–47.

32. T. Hu et al., "Testosterone-Associated Dietary Pattern Predicts Low Testosterone Levels and Hypogonadism," *Nutrients* 10, no. 11 (2018): 1786.

33. Wilson et al., "The Effects of Ketogenic Dieting."

34. K. Z. de Souza et al., "Efficacy of *Tribulus terrestris* for the Treatment of Hypoactive Sexual Desire Disorder in Postmenopausal Women: A Randomized, Double-Blinded, Placebo-Controlled Trial," *Menopause* 23, no. 11 (2016): 1252–56; F. B. C. Vale et al., "Efficacy of *Tribulus terrestris* for the Treatment of Premenopausal Women with Hypoactive Sexual Desire Disorder: A Randomized Double-Blinded, Placebo-Controlled Trial," *Gynecological Endocrinology.* 34, no. 5 (2018): 442–45; S. Palacios et al., "Effect of a Multi-Ingredient-Based Food Supplement on Sexual Function in Women with Low Sexual Desire," *BMC Women's Health: London* 19, no. 1 (2019): 58.

35. E. Steels et al., "Efficacy of a Proprietary Trigonella Foenum-Graecum L. Of-Husked Seed Extract in Reducing Menopausal Symptoms in Otherwise Healthy Women: A Double-Blind, Randomized, Placebo-Controlled Study," *Phytotherapy Research* 31, no. 9 (2017): 1316–22; S. Begum et al., "A Novel Extract of Fenugreek Husk (Fenusmart™) Alleviates Postmenopausal Symptoms and Helps to Establish the Hormonal Balance: A Randomized, Double-Blind, Placebo-Controlled Study," *Phytotherapy Research* 30, no. 11 (2016): 1775–84; A. Rao et al., "Influence of a Specialized Trigonella Foenum-Graecum Seed Extract (Libifem), on Testosterone, Estradiol, and Sexual Function in Healthy Menstruating Women: A Randomised Placebo-Controlled Study," *Phytotherapy Research* 29, no. 8 (2015): 1123–30.

36. de Souza et al., "Efficacy of *Tribulus terrestris*"; Vale et al., "Efficacy of *Tribulus terrestris*."

37. T. Takeuchi et al., "Serum Bisphenol A Concentrations Showed Gender Differences, Possibly Linked to Androgen Levels," *Biochemical and Biophysical Research Communications* 291, no. 1 (2002): 76–78; A. Tomza-Marciniak et al., "Effect of Bisphenol A on Reproductive Processes: A Review of In Vitro, In Vivo, and Epidemiological Studies," *Journal of Applied Toxicology* 38, no. 1 (2018): 51–80; Y. Hu et al., "The Association Between the Environmental Endocrine Disruptor Bisphenol A and Polycystic Ovary Syndrome: A Systematic Review and Meta-Analysis," *Gynecological Endocrinology* 34, no. 5 (2018): 370–77; A. Konieczna et al., "Serum Bisphenol A Concentrations Correlate with Serum Testosterone Levels in Women with Polycystic Ovary Syndrome," *Reproductive Toxicology* 82, no. 1 (2018): 32–37.

38. L. Le Corre et al., "BPA, an Energy Balance Disruptor," *Critical Reviews Food Science and Nutrition* 55, no. 6 (2015): 769–77; S. Legeay et al., "Is Bisphenol A an Environmental Obesogen?" *Fundamental & Clinical Pharmacology* 31, no. 6 (2017): 594–609; J. J. Heindel et al., "Environmental Obesogens: Mechanisms and Controversies," *Annual Review of Pharmacology Toxicology* 59, no. 1 (2019): 89–106; B. S. Rubin et al., "The Case for BPA as an Obesogen: Contributors to the Controversy," *Front Endocrinology (Lausanne)* 10, no. 30 (2019).

39. R. H. W. van Lunsen et al., "Maintaining Physiologic Testosterone Levels During Combined Oral Contraceptives by Adding Dehydroepiandrosterone: II. Effects on Sexual Function. A Phase II Randomized, Double-Blind, Placebo-Controlled Study," *Contraception* 98, no. 1 (2018): 56–62.

40. C. S. Scheffers et al., "Dehydroepiandrosterone for Women in the Peri- or Postmenopausal Phase," *Cochrane Database Systemic Reviews* 1 (2015).

## 4. THE KETO PARADOX

1. E. Vining et al., "A Multicenter Study of the Efficacy of the Ketogenic Diet," *Archives of Neurology* 55, no. 11 (1998): 1433–37; D. R. Nordli et al., "Experience with the Ketogenic Diet in Infants," *Pediatrics* 108, no. 1 (2001): 129–33; K. Tran et al., "Can You Predict an Immediate, Complete, and Sustained Response to the

Ketogenic Diet?" *Epilepsia* 46, no. 4 (2005): 580–82; E. Neal et al., "The Ketogenic Diet for the Treatment of Childhood Epilepsy: A Randomised Controlled Trial," *The Lancet Neurology* 7, no. 6 (2008): 500–506; L. Shah et al., "How Often Is Antiseizure Drug-Free Ketogenic Diet Therapy Achieved?" *Epilepsy & Behavior* 93, no. 1 (2019): 29–31; B. Gilbert, "Benefits and Complications of the Ketogenic Diet for Epilepsy," *Neurology Advisor,* https://www.neurologyadvisor.com/topics/epilepsy/benefits-and-complications-of-the-ketogenic-diet-for-epilepsy/. Accessed November 27, 2019.

2. T. J. W. McDonald et al., "Ketogenic Diets for Adult Neurological Disorders," *Neurotherapeutics* 15, no. 4 (2018): 1018–31; M. Rusek et al., "Ketogenic Diet in Alzheimer's Disease," *International Journal of Molecular Sciences* 20, no. 16 (2019): 3892; G. M. Broom et al., "The Ketogenic Diet as a Potential Treatment and Prevention Strategy for Alzheimer's Disease," *Nutrition* 60 (2019): 118–21; R. Nagpal et al., "Modified Mediterranean-Ketogenic Diet Modulates Gut Microbiome and Short-Chain Fatty Acids in Association with Alzheimer's Disease Markers in Subjects with Mild Cognitive Impairment," *EBioMedicine* 47 (2019): 529–42.

3. H. Y. Chung et al., "Rationale, Feasibility, and Acceptability of Ketogenic Diet for Cancer Treatment," *Journal of Cancer Prevention* 22, no. 3 (2017): 127–134; D. D. Weber et al., "Ketogenic Diet in the Treatment of Cancer—Where Do We Stand?" *Molecular Metabolism* 33 (2020): 102–21.

4. B. D. Hopkins et al., "Suppression of Insulin Feedback Enhances the Efficacy of PI3K Inhibitors," *Nature* 560, no. 7719 (2018): 499–503.

5. A. F. Luat et al., "The Ketogenic Diet: A Practical Guide for Pediatricians," *Pediatric Annals* 45, no. 12 (2016): e446–50; G. Muscogiuri et al., "The Management of Very Low-Calorie Ketogenic Diet in Obesity Outpatient Clinic: A Practical Guide," *Journal of Translational Medicine* 17, no. 1 (2019): 356.

6. A. Johannessen et al., "Prolactin, Growth Hormone, Thyrotropin, 3, 5, 3'-Triiodothyronine, and Thyroxine Responses to Exercise After Fat- and Carbohydrate-Enriched Diet," *The Journal of Clinical Endocrinology & Metabolism* 52, no. 1 (1981): 56–61; L. J. McCargar et al., "Dietary Carbohydrate-to-Fat Ratio: Influence on Whole-Body Nitrogen Retention, Substrate Utilization, and Hormone Response in Healthy Male Subjects," *The American Journal of Clinical Nutrition* 49, no. 6 (1989): 1169–78; J. Langfort et al., "Effect of Low-Carbohydrate-Ketogenic Diet on Metabolic and Hormonal Responses to Graded Exercise in Men," *Journal of Physiology and Pharmacology: An Official Journal of the Polish Physiological Society* 47, no. 2 (1996): 361–71; F. Q. Nuttall et al., "The Metabolic Response to a High-Protein, Low-Carbohydrate Diet in Men with Type 2 Diabetes Mellitus," *Metabolism* 55, no. 2 (2006): 243–51; A. E. Lima-Silva et al., "Low Carbohydrate Diet Affects the Oxygen Uptake on-Kinetics and Rating of Perceived Exertion in High-Intensity Exercise," *Psychophysiology* 48, no. 2 (2011): 277–84; A. Zajac et al., "The Effects of a Ketogenic Diet on Exercise Metabolism and Physical Performance in Off-Road Cyclists," *Nutrients* 6, no. 7 (2014): 2493–508; K. D. Hall et al., "Energy Expenditure and Body Composition Changes After an Isocaloric Ketogenic Diet

in Overweight and Obese Men," *The American Journal of Clinical Nutrition* 104, no. 2 (2016): 324–33; S. Vargas et al., "Efficacy of Ketogenic Diet on Body Composition During Resistance Training in Trained Men: A Randomized Controlled Trial," *Journal of the International Society of Sports Nutrition* 15, no. 1 (2018): 31.

7. A. M. Johnstone et al., "Effects of a High-Protein Ketogenic Diet on Hunger, Appetite, and Weight Loss in Obese Men Feeding Ad Libitum," *The American Journal of Clinical Nutrition* 87, no. 1 (2008): 44–55.

8. S. R. Nymo et al., "Timeline of Changes in Appetite During Weight Loss with a Ketogenic Diet," *International Journal of Obesity* 41, no. 8 (2017): 1224–31.

9. Hall et al., "Energy Expenditure and Body Composition."

10. Vargas et al., "Efficacy of Ketogenic Diet."

11. M. J. Sharman et al., "A Ketogenic Diet Favorably Affects Serum Biomarkers for Cardiovascular Disease in Normal-Weight Men," *The Journal of Nutrition* 132, no. 7 (2002): 1879–85.

12. K. K. Ryan et al., "Dietary Manipulations That Induce Ketosis Activate the HPA Axis in Male Rats and Mice: A Potential Role for Fibroblast Growth Factor-21," *Endocrinology* 159, no. 1 (2017): 400–413.

13. C. M. Young et al., "Effect on Body Composition and Other Parameters in Obese Young Men of Carbohydrate Level of Reduction Diet," *The American Journal of Clinical Nutrition* 24, no. 3 (1971): 290–96; S. B. Hulley et al., "Lipid and Lipoprotein Responses of Hypertriglyceridaemic Outpatients to a Low-Carbohydrate Modification of the AHA Fat-Controlled Diet," *The Lancet* 300, no. 7777 (1972): 551–55; B. Fagerberg et al., "Weight-Reducing Diets: Role of Carbohydrates on Sympathetic Nervous Activity and Hypotensive Response," *International Journal of Obesity* 8, no. 3 (1984): 237–43; J. W. Helge et al., "Prolonged Adaptation to Fat-Rich Diet and Training: Effects on Body Fat Stores and Insulin Resistance in Man," *International Journal of Obesity* 26, no. 8 (2002): 1118–24; J. S. Volek et al., "Body Composition and Hormonal Responses to a Carbohydrate-Restricted Diet," *Metabolism-Clinical and Experimental* 51, no. 7 (2002): 864–70; R. H. Stimson et al., "Dietary Macronutrient Content Alters Cortisol Metabolism Independently of Body Weight Changes in Obese Men," *The Journal of Clinical Endocrinology & Metabolism* 92, no. 11 (2007): 4480–84; A. R. Lane et al., "Influence of Dietary Carbohydrate Intake on the Free Testosterone: Cortisol Ratio Responses to Short-Term Intensive Exercise Training," *European Journal of Applied Physiology* 108, no. 6 (2010): 1125–31; K. Pilis et al., "Three-Year Chronic Consumption of Low-Carbohydrate Diet Impairs Exercise Performance and Has a Small Unfavorable Effect on Lipid Profile in Middle-Aged Men," *Nutrients* 10, no. 12 (2018): 1914; H. S. Waldman et al., "Effects of a 15-day Low Carbohydrate, High-Fat Diet in Resistance-Trained Men," *The Journal of Strength & Conditioning Research* 32, no. 11 (2018): 3103–11; M. M. Michalczyk et al., "Anaerobic Performance After a Low-Carbohydrate Diet (LCD) Followed by 7 Days of Carbohydrate Loading in Male Basketball Players," *Nutrients* 11, no. 4 (2019): 778.

14. L. Stern et al., "The Effects of Low-Carbohydrate Versus Conventional Weight

Loss Diets in Severely Obese Adults: One-Year Follow-Up of a Randomized Trial," *Annals of Internal Medicine* 140, no. 10 (2004): 778–85; I. Shai et al., "Weight Loss with a Low-Carbohydrate, Mediterranean, or Low-Fat Diet," *New England Journal of Medicine* 359, no. 3 (2008): 229–41; N. Iqbal et al., "Effects of a Low-Intensity Intervention That Prescribed a Low-Carbohydrate vs. a Low-Fat Diet in Obese, Diabetic Participants," *Obesity* 18, no. 9 (2010): 1733–38.

15. Volek et al., "Cardiovascular and Hormonal Aspects"; Volek et al., "Comparison of Energy-Restricted"; Dashti et al., "Long Term Effects of Ketogenic Diet"; Ruaño, "Physiogenomic Analysis of Weight Loss"; Durkalec-Michalski et al., "Effect of a Four-week Ketogenic Diet."

16. R. L. Williams et al., "Effectiveness of Weight Loss Interventions — Is there a Difference Between Men and Women? A Systematic Review," *Obesity Review* 16, no. 2 (2015): 171–86.

17. D. J. Millward et al., "Sex Differences in the Composition of Weight Gain and Loss in Overweight and Obese Adults," *British Journal of Nutrition* 111, no. 5 (2014): 933–43.

18. A. Wirth et al., "Gender Differences in Changes in Subcutaneous and Intra-Abdominal Fat During Weight Reduction: An Ultrasound Study," *Obesity Research* 6, no. 6 (1998): 393–99.

19. Men were 64 percent less likely to be aware of their weight ("weight perception"), 61 percent less likely to experience weight dissatisfaction, and 45 percent less likely to attempt weight loss. Men who attempted weight loss were 40 percent more likely than women to lose 10 pounds or more over one year, maintain that loss, and increase exercise. S. A. Tsai et al., "Gender Differences in Weight-Related Attitudes and Behaviors Among Overweight and Obese Adults in the United States," *American Journal of Men's Health* 10, no. 5 (2016): 389–98.

20. A. Furnham et al., "Body Image Dissatisfaction: Gender Differences in Eating Attitudes, Self-Esteem, and Reasons for Exercise," *Journal of Psychology* 136, no. 6 (2002): 581–96.

21. E. Johansson et al., "Obesity and Labour Market Success in Finland: The Difference Between Having a High BMI and Being Fat," *Economics and Human Biology* 7, no. 1 (2009): 36–45.

22. Diagnostic ranges for cortisol and blood glucose. I measure cortisol in blood and urine. I measure glucose in blood and the interstitial space with a continuous glucose monitor. This is how the American Diabetes Association defines prediabetes: borderline glycemia measured by any of three measures — fasting plasma glucose 100–125 mg/dL (5.6–6.9 mmol/L), 2-h plasma glucose 140–199 mg/dL (7.8–11.0 mmol/L), or hemoglobin A1c 5.7–6.4 percent (39–46 mmol/mol).

J. S. Yudkin, "'Prediabetes': Are There Problems with This Label? Yes, the Label Creates Further Problems!" *Diabetes Care* 39, no. 8 (2016): 1468–71; American Diabetes Association, "2. Classification and Diagnosis of Diabetes: Standards of Medical Care in Diabetes — 2018," *Diabetes Care* 41, no. 1 (2018): S13–27.

23. D. E. Laaksonen et al., "Serum Fatty Acid Composition Predicts Development

of Impaired Fasting Glycaemia and Diabetes in Middle-aged Men," *Diabetic Medicine* 19, no. 6 (2002): 456–64; R. M. Van Dam et al., "Dietary Fat and Meat Intake in Relation to Risk of Type 2 Diabetes in Men," *Diabetes Care* 25, no. 3 (2002): 417–24; G. Riccardi et al., "Dietary Fat, Insulin Sensitivity, and the Metabolic Syndrome," *Clinical Nutrition* 23, no. 4 (2004): 447–56; A. Shaheen et al., "A Hypothetical Model to Solve the Controversy over the Involvement of UCP2 in Palmitate-Induced β-cell Dysfunction," *Endocrine* 54, no. 2 (2016): 276–83; M. Mazidi et al., "Dietary Food Patterns and Glucose/Insulin Homeostasis: A Cross-sectional Study Involving 24,182 Adult Americans," *Lipids in Health and Disease* 16, no. 1 (2017): 192; M. Rapoport et al., "Triglycerides, Free Fatty Acids, and Glycemic Control: An Unresolved Puzzle," *The Israel Medical Association Journal* 20, no. 6 (2018): 385–87; A. Julibert et al., "Total and Subtypes of Dietary Fat Intake and Its Association with Components of the Metabolic Syndrome in a Mediterranean Population at High Cardiovascular Risk," *Nutrients* 11, no. 7 (2019): 1493.

24. J. Y. Lee et al., "Saturated Fatty Acids, but Not Unsaturated Fatty Acids, Induce the Expression of Cyclooxygenase-2 Mediated Through Toll-Like Receptor 4," *Journal of Biological Chemistry* 276, no. 20 (2001): 16683–89; J. M. Fernández-Real et al., "Insulin Resistance, Inflammation, and Serum Fatty Acid Composition." *Diabetes Care* 26, no. 5 (2003): 1362–68; K. M. Ajuwon et al., "Palmitate Activates the NF-κB Transcription Factor and Induces IL-6 and TNFα Expression in 3T3-L1 Adipocytes," *The Journal of Nutrition* 135, no. 8 (2005): 1841–46; C. Klein-Platat et al., "Plasma Fatty Acid Composition Is Associated with the Metabolic Syndrome and Low-Grade Inflammation in Overweight Adolescents," *The American Journal of Clinical Nutrition* 82, no. 6 (2005): 1178–84; A. R. Weatherill et al., "Saturated and Polyunsaturated Fatty Acids Reciprocally Modulate Dendritic Cell Functions Mediated Through TLR4," *The Journal of Immunology* 174, no. 9 (2005): 5390–97; S. Santos et al., "Systematic Review of Saturated Fatty Acids on Inflammation and Circulating Levels of Adipokines," *Nutrition Research* 33, no. 9 (2013): 687–95; J. E. Kaikkonen et al., "High Serum n6 Fatty Acid Proportion Is Associated with Lowered LDL Oxidation and Inflammation: The Cardiovascular Risk in Young Finns Study," *Free Radical Research* 48, no. 4 (2014): 420–26; C. Harris et al., "Associations Between Fatty Acids and Low-Grade Inflammation in Children from the MELISSAplus Birth Cohort Study," *European Journal of Clinical Nutrition* 71, no. 11 (2017): 1303–11; D. M. Rocha et al., "The Role of Dietary Fatty Acid Intake in Inflammatory Gene Expression: A Critical Review," *São Paulo Medical Journal* 135, no. 2 (2017): 157–68.

25. L. Arab et al., "Biomarkers and the Measurement of Fatty Acids," *Public Health Nutrition* 5, no. 6a (2002): 865–71; C. Kasapis et al., "The Effects of Physical Activity on Serum C-Reactive Protein and Inflammatory Markers: A Systematic Review," *Journal of the American College of Cardiology* 45, no. 10 (2005): 1563–69; M. Gleeson et al., "The Anti-Inflammatory Effects of Exercise: Mechanisms and Implications for the Prevention and Treatment of Disease," *Nature Reviews*

*Immunology* 11, no. 9 (2011): 607–15; B. Ruiz-Núñez et al., "Lifestyle and Nutritional Imbalances Associated with Western Diseases: Causes and Consequences of Chronic Systemic Low-Grade Inflammation in an Evolutionary Context," *The Journal of Nutritional Biochemistry* 24, no. 7 (2013): 1183–1201; S. Santos et al., "Fatty Acids Derived from a Food Frequency Questionnaire and Measured in the Erythrocyte Membrane in Relation to Adiponectin and Leptin Concentrations," *European Journal of Clinical Nutrition* 68, no. 5 (2014): 555–60; M. Mazidi et al., "Impact of the Dietary Fatty Acid Intake on C-Reactive Protein Levels in US Adults," *Medicine* 96, no. 7 (2017): e5736.

26. Rodrigues et al., "The Action of β-hydroxybutyrate."

27. G. Beccuti et al., "Sleep and Obesity," *Current Opinion in Clinical Nutrition and Metabolic Care* 14, no. 4 (2011): 402–12.

## 5. HOW TO START AND WHAT TO EAT

1. T. L. Stanley et al., "Effects of Growth Hormone–Releasing Hormone on Visceral Fat, Metabolic, and Cardiovascular Indices in Human Studies," *Growth Hormone & IGF Research* 25, no. 2 (2015): 59–65.

2. L. R. Squire et al., "Conscious and Unconscious Memory Systems," *Cold Spring Harbor Perspectives in Biology* 7, no. 3 (2015): a021667; J. Goodman et al., "Memory Systems and the Addicted Brain," *Frontiers in Psychiatry* 7 (2016): 24; M. M. Torregrossa et al., "Neuroscience of Learning and Memory for Addiction Medicine: From Habit Formation to Memory Reconsolidation," *Progress in Brain Research* 223 (2016): 91–113; J. Goodman et al., "The Dorsolateral Striatum Selectively Mediates Extinction of Habit Memory," *Neurobiology of Learning and Memory* 136 (2016): 54–62; L. Mang et al., "The Influence of Mood and Attitudes Towards Eating on Cognitive and Autobiographical Memory Flexibility in Female University Students," *Psychiatry Research* 269 (2018): 444–49.

3. E. Patrono et al., "Transitionality in Addiction: A 'Temporal Continuum' Hypotheses Involving the Aberrant Motivation, the Hedonic Dysregulation, and the Aberrant Learning," *Medical Hypotheses* 93 (2016): 62–70.

4. V. Voon, "Cognitive Biases in Binge Eating Disorder: The Hijacking of Decision Making," *CNS Spectrums* 20, no. 6 (2015): 566–73.

5. J. Goodman et al., "Enhancing and Impairing Extinction of Habit Memory Through Modulation of NMDA Receptors in the Dorsolateral Striatum," *Neuroscience* 352 (2017): 216–25.

6. Mang et al., "The Influence of Mood and Attitudes."

7. For whole foods, take total carbs and subtract fiber (in grams) to determine your net carbs. For processed food, subtract fiber (in grams) and sugar alcohol (in grams from total carbs in grams) to determine your net carbs.

8. Laboratory testing for insulin resistance involves both impaired fasting glucose and impaired glucose tolerance. These are the diagnostic criteria of optimal, borderline, prediabetes, and diabetes that I have used in my medical practice based on the best evidence, but you should know that numerous groups, from the

American Diabetes Association to the World Health Organization, use criteria that lack consensus.

- Fasting glucose: optimal 70–85, borderline 86–99, prediabetes 100–125, diabetes greater than 126 mg/dL
- Continuous glucose monitor with optimal average glucose less than 100 and standard deviation less than 15 mg/dL (in my opinion, based on clinical experience and my preferred way to diagnose insulin issues)
- 2-hour postprandial glucose prediabetes 140–199 mg/dL, diabetes greater than 199 mg/dL
- hemoglobin optimal less than 5 percent, borderline 5.0–5.6 percent, prediabetes A1C 5.7–6.4 percent, diabetes greater than 6.4 percent

World Health Organization, "Definition and Diagnosis of Diabetes Mellitus and Intermediate Hyperglycaemia: Report of a WHO/IDF Consultation" (2006): 1–50; N. Bansal, "Prediabetes Diagnosis and Treatment: A Review," *World Journal of Diabetes* 6, no. 2 (2015): 296; W. C. Y. Yip et al., "Prevalence of Pre-Diabetes Across Ethnicities: A Review of Impaired Fasting Glucose (IFG) and Impaired Glucose Tolerance (IGT) for Classification of Dysglycaemia," *Nutrients* 9, no. 11 (2017): 1273; Z. Punthakee et al., "Classification and Diagnosis of Diabetes, Prediabetes, and Metabolic Syndrome," *Canadian Journal of Diabetes* 42 (2018): S10–15; American Diabetes Association, "2. Classification and Diagnosis of Diabetes: Standards of Medical Care in Diabetes — 2018," *Diabetes Care* 41, no. 1 (2018): S13–27.

9. A. Hozawa et al., "Association Between Body Mass Index and All-Cause Death in Japanese Population: Pooled Individual Participant Data Analysis of 13 Cohort Studies," *Journal of Epidemiology* 29, no. 12 (2019): 457–63; M. D. Rahman et al., "Trend, Projection, and Appropriate Body Mass Index Cut-Off Point for Diabetes and Hypertension in Bangladesh," *Diabetes Research and Clinical Practice* 126 (2017): 43–53.

10. This online calculator is offered by the Centers for Disease Control: https://www.cdc.gov/healthyweight/assessing/bmi/adult_bmi/english_bmi_calculator/bmi_calculator.html, accessed May 20, 2020.

11. When I am coaching a patient about the Gottfried Protocol, I ask if they want the basic or the advanced approach. For people who have the bandwidth, it can be helpful to measure more advanced metrics, including the following:
- Daily fingerstick for blood sugar and ketones (see Resources for recommended brands, like Keto-mojo and Precision Extra), in order to calculate the glucose ketone index
- Continuous glucose monitor (see Resources for recommended brands)
- Bluetooth body composition scale (see Resources — I use Renpho.)
- Resting metabolic rate
- Exercise performance, such as VO2 max

12. One of the best descriptions of the ketogenic ratio is in this book: Jacob Wilson and Ryan Lowery, *The Ketogenic Bible* (Las Vegas: Victory Belt, 2017), 39–40.

13. Proteins are mixed in their ketogenic effect. Why? Some building blocks of protein, called amino acids, are ketogenic and others are anti-ketogenic. Examples of ketogenic amino acids are leucine and lysine. An example of an anti-ketogenic amino acid is alanine.

14. I. A. Cohen, "A Model for Determining Total Ketogenic Ratio (TKR) for Evaluating the Ketogenic Property of a Weight-Reduction Diet," *Medical Hypotheses* 73, no. 3 (2009): 377–81.

15. Young et al., "Effect on Body Composition."

16. S. H. Duncan et al., "Reduced Dietary Intake of Carbohydrates by Obese Subjects Results in Decreased Concentrations of Butyrate and Butyrate-Producing Bacteria in Feces," *Applied and Environmental Microbiology* 73, no. 4 (2007): 1073–78.

17. To calculate the net carbs in processed foods, subtract the fiber and a portion of the sugar alcohols. So for one-third of a medium avocado, that's 4 grams of carbohydrates, less 3 grams of fiber (4g – 3 g = 1 g), so 1 net carbohydrate. For my favorite brownies, which I recommend in Resources, that's 13 total carbs per each serving of brownie, less 5 grams of fiber, less 7 grams of sugar alcohols (in this case, erythritol and allulose), or 1 net carb.

18. J. Rehm et al., "Alcohol Use and Cancer in the European Union," *European Addiction Research* (2020): 1–8; S. Parida et al., "Microbial Alterations and Risk Factors of Breast Cancer: Connections and Mechanistic Insights," *Cells* 9, no. 5 (2020): 1091.

19. X. Yao et al., "Change in Moderate Alcohol Consumption and Quality of Life: Evidence from 2 Population-Based Cohorts," *CMAJ* 191, no. 27 (2019): E753–60.

20. M. Venkatesh et al., "Dietary Oil Composition Differentially Modulates Intestinal Endotoxin Transport and Postprandial Endotoxemia," *Nutrition & Metabolism* 10, no. 1 (2013): 6.

21. A. Dagfinn et al., "Nut Consumption and Risk of Cardiovascular Disease, Total Cancer, All-Cause and Cause-Specific Mortality: A Systematic Review and Dose-Response Meta-Analysis of Prospective Studies," *BMC Medicine* 14, no. 1 (2016): 207; C. Guo-Chong et al., "Nut Consumption in Relation to All-Cause and Cause-Specific Mortality: A Meta-Analysis 18 Prospective Studies," *Food & Function* 8, no. 11 (2017): 3893–905.

22. M. P. St-Onge et al., "Consumption of a Functional Oil Rich in Phytosterols and Medium-Chain Triglyceride Oil Improves Plasma Lipid Profiles in Men," *The Journal of Nutrition* 133, no. 6, (2003): 1815–20; J. R. Han et al., "Effects of Dietary Medium-Chain Triglyceride on Weight Loss and Insulin Sensitivity in a Group of Moderately Overweight Free-Living Type 2 Diabetic Chinese Subjects," *Metabolism* 56, no. 7 (2007): 985–91; M. P. St-Onge et al., "Medium-Chain Triglyceride Oil Consumption as Part of a Weight Loss Diet Does Not Lead to an Adverse Metabolic Profile When Compared to Olive Oil," *Journal of the American College of Nutrition* 27, no. 5 (2008): 547–52.

23. K. Mumme et al., "Effects of Medium-Chain Triglycerides on Weight Loss and

Body Composition: A Meta-Analysis of Randomized Controlled Trials," *Journal of the Academy of Nutrition and Dietetics* 115, no. 2 (2015): 249–63.

24. T. Maher et al., "A Comparison of the Satiating Properties of Medium-Chain Triglycerides and Conjugated Linoleic Acid in Participants with Healthy Weight and Overweight or Obesity," *European Journal of Nutrition* (2020): 1–13.

25. Here are additional details about MCT.

MCT oil increases ketones by 19 percent and can help flip the metabolic switch from burning glucose to burning fat. (C. Vandenberghe et al., "Medium-Chain Triglycerides Modulate the Ketogenic Effect of a Metabolic Switch," *Frontiers in Nutrition* 7 (2020): 3–6.

Additionally, in limited studies in Alzheimer's disease, some measures of cognition improved with addition of MCT oil to the diet (K. I. Avgerinos et al., "Medium-Chain Triglycerides Induce Mild Ketosis and May Improve Cognition in Alzheimer's Disease: A Systematic Review and Meta-Analysis of Human Studies," *Ageing Research Reviews* [2019]: 101,001), and brain utilization of ketones may double (E. Croteau et al., "Ketogenic Medium-Chain Triglycerides Increase Brain Energy Metabolism in Alzheimer's Disease," *Journal of Alzheimer's Disease* 64, no. 2 [2018]: 551–61).

MCT talks to hormones too and may help you become more insulin sensitive and lower your adiponectin within six weeks, at least according to one small uncontrolled study (D. D. Thomas et al., "Effects of Medium-Chain Triglycerides Supplementation on Insulin Sensitivity and Beta Cell Function: A Feasibility Study," *PLoS One* 14, no. 12 (2019).

26. The mechanism for damage is believed to be through the elevation of bacterial toxins from the gut, known as endotoxemia, for five to eight hours after you eat it. P. Dandona et al., "Macronutrient Intake Induces Oxidative and Inflammatory Stress: Potential Relevance to Atherosclerosis and Insulin Resistance," *Experimental & Molecular Medicine* 42, no. 4 (2010): 245–53; F. Biobaku et al., "Macronutrient-Mediated Inflammation and Oxidative Stress: Relevance to Insulin Resistance, Obesity, and Atherogenesis," *The Journal of Clinical Endocrinology & Metabolism* 104, no. 12 (2019): 6118–28.

27. When you eat saturated or trans fats together with refined carbohydrates, the mechanism for damage is a combination of oxidative stress, unresolved inflammation, endotoxemia, increased expression of SOCS-3 and TLR4, blocking IRS-1 and PI3K pathways inducing insulin resistance, according to personal communication with Mark Houston, MD, and Dandona et al., "Macronutrient Intake."

28. Y. Bao et al., "Association of Nut Consumption with Total and Cause-Specific Mortality," *The New England Journal of Medicine* 369, no. 21 (2013): 2001–11.

29. C. Smith-Spangler et al., "Are Organic Foods Safer or Healthier Than Conventional Alternatives? A Systematic Review," *Annals of Internal Medicine* 157, no. 5 (2012): 343–66; S. Watson, "Organic Food No More Nutritious Than Conventionally Grown Food," *Harvard Women's Health Watch,* September 5, 2012,

https://www.health.harvard.edu/blog/organic-foodno-more-nutritious-than-conventionally-grown-food-201209055264. Accessed May 6, 2020.

30. A. S. Abargouei et al., "Effect of Dairy Consumption on Weight and Body Composition in Adults: A Systematic Review and Meta-Analysis of Randomized Controlled Clinical Trials," *International Journal of Obesity* 36, no. 12 (2012): 1485–93.

31. California Avocados, "Avocado Nutritional Information," https://www.californiaavocado.com/nutrition/nutrients. Accessed May 6, 2020.

32. S. Kim et al., "Effects of Growth Hormone on Glucose Metabolism and Insulin Resistance in Humans," *Annals of Pediatric Endocrinology & Metabolism* 22, no. 3 (2017): 145.

33. L. A. Frohman, "Growth Hormone," *Encyclopedia of Neuroscience,* vol. 1 (London: Academic Press, 2009).

34. Diabetes Teaching Center at the University of California, San Francisco, "Blood Sugar & Other Hormones," https://dtc.ucsf.edu/types-of-diabetes/type1/understanding-type-1-diabetes/how-the-body-processes-sugar/blood-sugar-other-hormones/

35. R. Lanzi et al., "Elevated Insulin Levels Contribute to the Reduced Growth Hormone (GH) Response to GH-Releasing Hormone in Obese Subjects," *Metabolism* 48, no. 9 (1999): 1152–56; J. Xu et al., "Crosstalk Between Growth Hormone and Insulin Signaling," *Vitamins & Hormones* 80 (2009): 125–53; H. Qiu et al., "Influence of Insulin on Growth Hormone Secretion, Level, and Growth Hormone Signaling," *Sheng Li Xue Bao* 69, no. 5 (2017): 541–56.

36. M. La Merrill et al., "Toxicological Function of Adipose Tissue: Focus on Persistent Organic Pollutants," *Environmental Health Perspectives* 121, no. 2 (2013): 162–69.

37. Your liver processes toxins in two phases. In phase one, it converts fat-soluble toxins into water-soluble substances. At the end of phase two, the liver excretes these water-soluble toxins via urine, stool, sweat, and other body fluids. In a detoxification protocol, this two-step process needs to be managed in the opposite order: optimize phase two before triggering phase one. This is one of the reasons why detoxification and "cleanse" programs are controversial and can make people sick; if toxins are removed from tissues at a higher rate than they are removed from the body, it makes a person feel terrible and can even have severe consequences. Think of it this way: you don't warm up the car in the garage, and then open the garage door to let out the fumes.

38. J. Obert et al., "Popular Weight Loss Strategies: A Review of Four Weight Loss Techniques," *Current Gastroenterology Reports* 19, no. 12 (2017): 61.

39. M. S. Duchowny, "Food for Thought: The Ketogenic Diet and Adverse Effects in Children," *Epilepsy Currents* 5, no. 4 (2005): 152–54.

40. G. Zong et al., "Consumption of Meals Prepared at Home and Risk of Type 2 Diabetes: An Analysis of Two Prospective Cohort Studies," *PLoS Medicine* 13, no. 7 (2016): e1002052.

## 6. DETOXING, CIRCADIAN FASTING, AND TROUBLESHOOTING

1. M. M. Hetherington et al., "Understanding the Science of Portion Control and the Art of Downsizing," *Proceedings of the Nutrition Society* 77, no. 3 (2018): 347–55.

2. J. J. Meidenbauer et al., "The Glucose Ketone Index Calculator: A Simple Tool to Monitor Therapeutic Efficacy for Metabolic Management of Brain Cancer," *Nutrition & Metabolism* 12, no. 1 (2015): 1–7.

3. Y. Li, "Exogenous Stimuli Maintain Intraepithelial Lymphocytes Via Aryl Hydrocarbon Receptor Activation," *Cell* 147, no. 3 (2011): 629–40.

4. A. Paoli et al., "Effect of Ketogenic Mediterranean Diet with Phytoextracts and Low Carbohydrates/High-Protein Meals on Weight, Cardiovascular Risk Factors, Body Composition, and Diet Compliance in Italian Council Employees," *Nutrition Journal* 10, no. 1 (2011): 112; A. Paoli et al., "Long Term Successful Weight Loss with a Combination Biphasic Ketogenic Mediterranean Diet and Mediterranean Diet Maintenance Protocol," *Nutrients* 5, no. 12 (2013): 5205–17; A. Paoli et al., "Ketogenic Diet and Phytoextracts," *Scientific Advisory Board* 21, no. 4 (2010): 24–29; A. Paoli et al., "Ketogenic Diet Does Not Affect Strength Performance in Elite Artistic Gymnasts," *Journal of the International Society of Sports Nutrition* 9, no. 1 (2012): 34; A. Paoli et al., "Effects of n-3 Polyunsaturated Fatty Acids (ω-3) Supplementation on Some Cardiovascular Risk Factors with a Ketogenic Mediterranean Diet," *Marine Drugs* 13, no. 2 (2015): 996–1009; G. Bosco et al., "Effects of the Ketogenic Diet in Overweight Divers Breathing Enriched Air Nitrox," *Scientific Reports* 8, no. 1 (2018): 1–8; A. Paoli et al., "Effects of a Ketogenic Diet in Overweight Women with Polycystic Ovary Syndrome," *Journal of Translational Medicine* 18, no. 1 (2020): 1–11.

5. Y. Aitbali et al., "Glyphosate Based-Herbicide Exposure Affects Gut Microbiota, Anxiety, and Depression-Like Behaviors in Mice," *Neurotoxicology and Teratology* (2018); I. Argou-Cardozo et al., "Clostridium Bacteria and Autism Spectrum Conditions: A Systematic Review and Hypothetical Contribution of Environmental Glyphosate Levels," *Medical Sciences* 6, no. 2 (2018): 29; C. E. Gallegos et al., "Perinatal Glyphosate-Based Herbicide Exposure in Rats Alters Brain Antioxidant Status, Glutamate and Acetylcholine Metabolism, and Affects Recognition Memory," *Neurotoxicity Research* (2018): 1–12; P. Good. "Evidence the US Autism Epidemic Initiated by Acetaminophen (Tylenol) Is Aggravated by Oral Antibiotic Amoxicillin/Clavulanate (Augmentin) and Now Exponentially by Herbicide Glyphosate (Roundup)," *Clinical Nutrition ESPEN* 23 (2018): 171–83; L. N. Nielsen et al., "Glyphosate Has Limited Short-Term Effects on Commensal Bacterial Community Composition in the Gut Environment Due to Sufficient Aromatic Amino Acid Levels," *Environmental Pollution* 233 (2018): 364–76.

6. J. J. Gildea et al., "Protection Against Gluten-Mediated Tight Junction Injury with a Novel Lignite Extract Supplement," *Journal of Nutrition & Food Sciences* 6, no. 547 (2016): 2; J. J. Gildea et al., "Protective Effects of Lignite Extract Supplement

on Intestinal Barrier Function in Glyphosate-Mediated Tight Junction Injury," *Journal of Clinical Nutrition & Dietetics* 3, no. 1 (2017).

7. A. Di Ciaula et al., "Diet and Contaminants: Driving the Rise to Obesity Epidemics?" *Current Medicinal Chemistry* 26, no. 19 (2019): 3471–82; L. A. Hoepner, "Bisphenol A: A Narrative Review of Prenatal Exposure Effects on Adipogenesis and Childhood Obesity Via Peroxisome Proliferator-Activated Receptor Gamma," *Environmental Research* 173 (2019): 54–68; Rubin et al., "The Case for BPA as an Obesogen"; R. Chamorro-Garcia et al., "Current Research Approaches and Challenges in the Obesogen Field," *Frontiers in Endocrinology* 10 (2019): 167; J. J. Heindel, "History of the Obesogen Field: Looking Back to Look Forward," *Frontiers in Endocrinology* 10 (2019): 14.

8. K. Katoh et al., "Suppressing Effects of Bisphenol A on the Secretory Function of Ovine Anterior Pituitary Cells," *Cell Biology International* 28, no. 6 (2004): 463–69.

9. A. B. Javurek et al., "Effects of Exposure to Bisphenol A and Ethinyl Estradiol on the Gut Microbiota of Parents and Their Offspring in a Rodent Model," *Gut Microbes* 7, no. 6 (2016): 471–85; J. Xu et al., "Developmental Bisphenol A Exposure Modulates Immune-Related Diseases," *Toxics* 4, no. 4 (2016): 23; K. P. Lai et al., "Bisphenol A Alters Gut Microbiome: Comparative Metagenomics Analysis," *Environmental Pollution* 218 (2016): 923–30; L. Reddivari et al., "Perinatal Bisphenol A Exposure Induces Chronic Inflammation in Rabbit Offspring via Modulation of Gut Bacteria and Their Metabolites," *MSystems* 2, no. 5 (2017); Y. Malaisé et al., "Gut Dysbiosis and Impairment of Immune System Homeostasis in Perinatally Exposed Mice to Bisphenol A Precede Obese Phenotype Development," *Scientific Reports* 7, no. 1 (2017): 1–12; J. A. DeLuca et al., "Bisphenol-A Alters Microbiota Metabolites Derived from Aromatic Amino Acids and Worsens Disease Activity During Colitis," *Experimental Biology and Medicine* 243, no. 10 (2018): 864–75; T. R. Catron et al., " Host Developmental Toxicity of BPA and BPA Alternatives Is Inversely Related to Microbiota Disruption in Zebrafish," *Toxicological Sciences* 167, no. 2 (2019): 468–83.

10. K. Oishi, "Effect of Probiotics, Bifidobacterium Breve, and Lactobacillus Casei on Bisphenol A Exposure in Rats," *Bioscience, Biotechnology, and Biochemistry* 72, no. 6 (2008): 1409–15; S. Song et al., "The Anti-Allergic Activity of Lactobacillus Plantarum L67 and Its Application to Yogurt," *Journal of Dairy Science* 99, no. 12 (2016): 9372–82.

11. A. A. Ismail et al., "Chronic Magnesium Deficiency and Human Disease: Time for Reappraisal?" *QJM: An International Journal of Medicine* 111, no. 11 (2018): 759–63; M. S. Razzaque, "Magnesium: Are We Consuming Enough?" *Nutrients* 10, no. 12 (2018): 1863; J. L. Workinger et al., "Challenges in the Diagnosis of Magnesium Status," *Nutrients* 10, no. 9 (2018): 1202.

12. For a list of functional medicine clinicians, go to the "find a practitioner" link at the Institute of Functional Medicine, https://www.ifm.org/find-a-practitioner/. Accessed December 16, 2020.

13. J. Hussain et al., "Clinical Effects of Regular Dry Sauna Bathing: A Systematic Review," *Evidence-Based Complementary and Alternative Medicine* (2018).

14. C. P. Oliveira et al., "N-Acetylcysteine and/or Ursodeoxycholic Acid Associated with Metformin in Non-Alcoholic Steatohepatitis: An Open-Label Multicenter Randomized Controlled Trial," *Arquivos de Gastroenterologia* 56, no. 2 (2019): 184–90; D. Thakker et al., "N-Acetylcysteine for Polycystic Ovary Syndrome: A Systematic Review and Meta-Analysis of Randomized Controlled Clinical Trials," *Obstetrics and Gynecology International* (2015).

15. A. M. Fulghesu et al., "N-Acetyl-Cysteine Treatment Improves Insulin Sensitivity in Women with Polycystic Ovary Syndrome," *Fertility and Sterility* 77, no. 6 (2002): 1128–35; G. Oner et al., "Clinical, Endocrine, and Metabolic Effects of Metformin vs. N-acetyl-cysteine in Women with Polycystic Ovary Syndrome," *European Journal of Obstetrics & Gynecology and Reproductive Biology* 159, no. 1 (2011): 127–31.

16. A. Elnashar et al., "N-Acetyl Cysteine vs. Metformin in Treatment of Clomiphene Citrate–Resistant Polycystic Ovary Syndrome: A Prospective Randomized Controlled Study," *Fertility and Sterility* 88, no. 2 (2007): 406–9.

17. S. Ebrahimpour-Koujan et al., "Lower Glycemic Indices and Lipid Profile Among Type 2 Diabetes Mellitus Patients Who Received Novel Dose of Silybum Marianum (L.) Gaertn.(silymarin) Extract Supplement: A Triple-Blinded Randomized Controlled Clinical Trial," *Phytomedicine* 44 (2018): 39–44.

18. S. Rahmani et al., "Treatment of Non-Alcoholic Fatty Liver Disease with Curcumin: A Randomized Placebo-Controlled Trial," *Phytotherapy Research* 30, no. 9 (2016): 1540–48; Y. Panahi et al., "Efficacy and Safety of Phytosomal Curcumin in Non-Alcoholic Fatty Liver Disease: A Randomized Controlled Trial," *Drug Research* 67, no. 04 (2017): 244–51; R. Goodarzi et al., "Does Turmeric/Curcumin Supplementation Improve Serum Alanine Aminotransferase and Aspartate Aminotransferase Levels in Patients with Nonalcoholic Fatty Liver Disease? A Systematic Review and Meta-Analysis of Randomized Controlled Trials," *Phytotherapy Research* 33, no. 3 (2019): 561–70; F. Mansour-Ghanaei et al., "Efficacy of Curcumin/Turmeric on Liver Enzymes in Patients with Non-Alcoholic Fatty Liver Disease: A Systematic Review of Randomized Controlled Trials," *Integrative Medicine Research* 8, no. 1 (2019): 57–61; A. Ghaffari et al., "Turmeric and Chicory Seed Have Beneficial Effects on Obesity Markers and Lipid Profile in Non-Alcoholic Fatty Liver Disease (NAFLD)," *International Journal for Vitamin and Nutrition Research* (2019).

19. K. Gabel et al., "Effects of 8-hour Time Restricted Feeding on Body Weight and Metabolic Disease Risk Factors in Obese Adults: A Pilot Study," *Nutrition and Healthy Aging* 4, no. 4 (2018): 345–53, https://content.iospress.com/articles/nutrition-and-healthy-aging/nha170036.

20. M. N. Harvie, "The Effects of Intermittent or Continuous Energy Restriction on Weight Loss and Metabolic Disease Risk Markers: A Randomized Trial in Young Overweight Women," *International Journal of Obesity (London)* 35 (2011): 714–27;

S. Gil et al., "A Smartphone App Reveals Diurnal Eating Patterns in Humans That Can Be Modulated for Health Benefits," *Cell Metabolism* 22, no. 5 (2015): 789–98; G. M. Tinsley et al., "Effects of Intermittent Fasting on Body Composition."

21. A. Chaix et al., "The Effects of Time-Restricted Feeding on Lipid Metabolism and Adiposity," *Adipocyte* 4, no. 4 (2015): 319–24; H. Chung et al., "Time-Restricted Feeding Improves Insulin Resistance and Hepatic Steatosis in a Mouse Model of Postmenopausal Obesity," *Metabolism-Clinical and Experimental* 65, no. 12 (2016): 1743–54.

22. A. Chaix et al., "Time-Restricted Feeding Is a Preventative and Therapeutic Intervention Against Diverse Nutritional Challenges," *Cell Metabolism* 20, no. 6 (2014): 991–1005; R. Antoni et al., "Effects of Intermittent Fasting on Glucose and Lipid Metabolism," *Proceedings of the Nutrition Society* 76, no. 3 (2017): 361–68.

23. G. C. Melkani et al., "Time Restricted Feeding for Prevention and Treatment of Cardiometabolic Disorders," *The Journal of Physiology* 595, no. 12 (2017): 3691–700.

24. R. E. Patterson et al., "Intermittent Fasting and Human Metabolic Health," *Journal of the Academy of Nutrition and Dietetics* 115, no. 8 (2015): 1203–12; C. R. Marinac et al., "Prolonged Nightly Fasting and Breast Cancer Prognosis," *JAMA Oncology* 2, no. 8 (2016): 1049–55; L. A. Smith et al., "Translating Mechanism-Based Strategies to Break the Obesity–Cancer Link: A Narrative Review," *Journal of the Academy of Nutrition and Dietetics* 118, no. 4 (2018): 652–67.

25. E. N. Manoogian et al., "Circadian Rhythms, Time-Restricted Feeding, and Healthy Aging," *Ageing Research Reviews* 39 (2017): 59–67.

26. J. T. Haas et al., "Fasting the Microbiota to Improve Metabolism?" *Cell Metabolism* 26, no. 4 (2017): 584–85; R. Kivelä et al., "White Adipose Tissue Coloring by Intermittent Fasting," *Cell Research* 27, no. 11 (2017): 1300–1301; G. Li et al., "Intermittent Fasting Promotes White Adipose Browning and Decreases Obesity by Shaping the Gut Microbiota," *Cell Metabolism* 26, no. 4 (2017): 672–85.

27. S. Eslami et al., "Annual Fasting; The Early Calories Restriction for Cancer Prevention," *BioImpacts: BI* 2, no. 4 (2012): 213–15; A. Zarrinpar et al., "Diet and Feeding Pattern Affect the Diurnal Dynamics of the Gut Microbiome," *Cell Metabolism* 20, no. 6 (2014): 1006–17; A. Chaix et al. "The Effects of Time-Restricted Feeding"; J. L. Kaczmarek et al., "Complex Interactions of Circadian Rhythms, Eating Behaviors, and the Gastrointestinal Microbiota and Their Potential Impact on Health," *Nutrition Reviews* 75, no. 9 (2017): 673–82; Li et al., "Intermittent Fasting Promotes White"; R. E. Patterson et al., "Metabolic Effects of Intermittent Fasting." *Annual Review of Nutrition* 37 (2017): 371–93; E. Beli et al., "Restructuring of the Gut Microbiome by Intermittent Fasting Prevents Retinopathy and Prolongs Survival in db/db Mice," *Diabetes* (2018): db180158.

28. S. Panda, "Circadian Physiology of Metabolism." *Science* 354, no. 6315 (2016): 1008–15.

29. M. P. Mattson et al., "Impact of Intermittent Fasting on Health and Disease Pro-

cesses," *Ageing Research Reviews* 39 (2017): 46–58; B. K. Shin et al., "Intermittent Fasting Protects Against the Deterioration of Cognitive Function, Energy Metabolism, and Dyslipidemia in Alzheimer's Disease-Induced Estrogen Deficient Rats," *Experimental Biology and Medicine* 234, no. 4 (2018): 334–43.

30. M. Hatori et al., "Time-Restricted Feeding Without Reducing Caloric Intake Prevents Metabolic Diseases in Mice Fed a High-Fat Diet," *Cell Metabolism* 15, no. 6 (2012): 848–60.

31. K. M. Pursey et al., "Neural Responses to Visual Food Cues According to Weight Status: A Systematic Review of Functional Magnetic Resonance Imaging Studies," *Frontiers in Nutrition* 1 (2017): 7–18.

32. I learned this hack from Jeffrey Becker, MD, in a lecture he gave at the Integrative Psychiatry Institute, where I am on the faculty. He recommends 1 teaspoon of MCT oil at work, or half a nutrition bar, in the afternoon to help prevent cravings for alcohol.

33. M. C. Houston, "Treatment of Hypertension with Nutraceuticals, Vitamins, Antioxidants, and Minerals," *Expert Review of Cardiovascular Therapy* 5, no. 4 (2007): 681–91; S. T. Sinatra et al., *Nutritional and Integrative Strategies in Cardiovascular Medicine* (Boca Raton, FL: CRC Press, 2015); L. Rochette et al., "Alpha-Lipoic Acid: Molecular Mechanisms and Therapeutic Potential in Diabetes," *Canadian Journal of Physiology and Pharmacology* 93, no. 12 (2015): 1021–27; S. Kucukgoncu et al., "Alpha-Lipoic Acid (ALA) as a Supplementation for Weight Loss: Results from a Meta-Analysis of Randomized Controlled Trials," *Obesity Reviews* 18, no. 5 (2017): 594–601.

34. Rochette et al., "Alpha-Lipoic Acid."

35. K. H. Weylandt et al., "Omega-3 Fatty Acids and Their Lipid Mediators: Towards an Understanding of Resolvin and Protectin Formation," *Prostaglandins & Other Lipid Mediators* 97, nos. 3–4 (2012): 73–82; R. Ramaswami et al., "Fish Oil Supplementation in Pregnancy," *New England Journal of Medicine* 375, no. 26 (2016): 2599–601.

36. Yang et al., "Ratio of N-3/N-6 PUFAs"; C. J. Fabian et al., "Omega-3 Fatty Acids for Breast Cancer Prevention and Survivorship," *Breast Cancer Research* 17, no. 1 (2015): 1–11.

37. M. Houston, *Personalized and Precision Integrative Cardiovascular Medicine* (Philadelphia: Lippincott Williams & Wilkins, 2019); Z. Ilyas et al., "The Effect of Berberine on Weight Loss in Order to Prevent Obesity: A Systematic Review," *Biomedicine & Pharmacotherapy* 127 (2020): 110137; M. Rondanelli et al., "Polycystic Ovary Syndrome Management: A Review of the Possible Amazing Role of Berberine," *Archives of Gynecology and Obstetrics* (2020): 1–8.

38. C. N. Serhan, "Pro-Resolving Lipid Mediators Are Leads for Resolution Physiology," *Nature* 510, no. 7503 (2014): 92–101; C. N. Serhan et al., "Resolvins in Inflammation: Emergence of the Pro-Resolving Superfamily of Mediators," *The Journal of Clinical Investigation* 128, no. 7 (2018): 2657–69; P. C. Norris et al., "Identification of Specialized Pro-Resolving Mediator Clusters from Healthy Adults After

Intravenous Low-Dose Endotoxin and Omega-3 Supplementation: A Method-
ological Validation," *Scientific Reports* 8, no. 1 (2018): 1–13.

39. C. C. Douglas et al., "Role of Diet in the Treatment of Polycystic Ovary Syndrome," *Fertility and Sterility* 85, no. 3 (2006): 679–88; Gottfried, *The Hormone
Cure,* M. McGrice et al., "The Effect of Low Carbohydrate Diets on Fertility Hormones and Outcomes in Overweight and Obese Women: A Systematic Review,"
*Nutrients* 9, no. 3 (2017): 204; L. Barrea et al., "Source and Amount of Carbohydrate in the Diet and Inflammation in Women with Polycystic Ovary Syndrome,"
*Nutrition Research Reviews* 31, no. 2 (2018): 291–301; L. Barrea et al., "Adherence
to the Mediterranean Diet, Dietary Patterns, and Body Composition in Women
with Polycystic Ovary Syndrome (PCOS)," *Nutrients* 11, no. 10 (2019): 2278.

40. Mavropoulos et al., "The Effects of a Low-Carbohydrate"; Gottfried, *The Hor-
mone Cure;* D. Kulak et al., "Should the Ketogenic Diet Be Considered for En-
hancing Fertility?" *Maturitas* 74, no. 1 (2013): 10–13; Muscogiuri et al., "Current
Insights into Inositol Isoforms"; M. Melanie et al., "The Effect of Low Carbo-
hydrate Diets on Fertility Hormones and Outcomes in Overweight and Obese
Women: A Systematic Review," *Nutrients* 9, no. 3 (2017): 204; M. Caprio et al.,
"Very-Low-Calorie Ketogenic Diet (VLCKD) in the Management of Metabolic
Diseases: Systematic Review and Consensus Statement from the Italian Society of
Endocrinology (SIE)," *Journal of Endocrinological Investigation* 42, no. 11 (2019):
1365–86; Paoli et al., "Effects of a Ketogenic Diet in Overweight Women."

41. Gottfried, *The Hormone Cure;* M. J. Carvalho et al., "Controversial Association
Between Polycystic Ovary Syndrome and Breast Cancer," *European Journal of
Obstetrics & Gynecology and Reproductive Biology* 243 (2019): 125–32.

42. A. Balen, "Polycystic Ovary Syndrome and Cancer," *Human Reproduction Update*
7, no. 6 (2001): 522–25; Gottfried, *The Hormone Cure;* C. C. Shen et al., "A Nationwide Population-Based Retrospective Cohort Study of the Risk of Uterine, Ovarian, and Breast Cancer in Women with Polycystic Ovary Syndrome," *The Oncologist* 20, no. 1 (2015): 45; F. Shobeiri et al., "The Association Between Polycystic
Ovary Syndrome and Breast Cancer: A Meta-Analysis," *Obstetrics & Gynecology
Science* 59, no. 5 (2016): 367–72.

43. Gottfried, *The Hormone Cure;* J. Barry et al., "Risk of Endometrial, Ovarian, and
Breast Cancer in Women with Polycystic Ovary Syndrome: A Systematic Review
and Meta-Analysis," *Human Reproduction Update* 20, no. 5 (2014): 748–58; M.
Gottschau et al., "Risk of Cancer Among Women with Polycystic Ovary Syndrome: A Danish Cohort Study." *Gynecologic Oncology* 136, no. 1 (2015): 99–103;
H. R. Harris et al., "Polycystic Ovary Syndrome and Risk of Endometrial, Ovarian, and Breast Cancer: A Systematic Review," *Fertility Research and Practice* 2,
no. 1 (2016): 14; D. C. Ding et al., "Association Between Polycystic Ovarian Syndrome and Endometrial, Ovarian, and Breast Cancer: A Population-Based Cohort Study in Taiwan," *Medicine* 97, no. 39 (2018).

44. Gottfried, *The Hormone Cure;* Barry et al., "Risk of Endometrial, Ovarian, and
Breast Cancer"; Shen et al., "A Nationwide Population-Based Retrospective";

Gottschau et al., "Risk of Cancer Among Women"; Harris et al., "Polycystic Ovary Syndrome"; Ding et al., "Association Between Polycystic Ovarian Syndrome."

## 7. TRANSITION

1. R. R. Wing et al., "Weight Gain at the Time of Menopause," *Archives of Internal Medicine* 151, no. 1 (1991): 97–102; G. M. Van Dijk et al., "The Association Between Vasomotor Symptoms and Metabolic Health in Peri- and Postmenopausal Women: A Systematic Review," *Maturitas* 80, no. 2 (2015): 140–47; P. Tuomikoski et al., "Vasomotor Symptoms and Metabolic Syndrome," *Maturitas* 97 (2017): 61–65; S. Sayan et al., "Relationship Between Vasomotor Symptoms and Metabolic Syndrome in Postmenopausal Women," *Journal of International Medical Research* 46, no. 10 (2018): 4157–66.

2. V. D. Longo et al., "Fasting, Circadian Rhythms, and Time-Restricted Feeding in Healthy Lifespan," *Cell Metabolism* 23, no. 6 (2016): 1048–59.

3. F. Coucke, "Food Intolerance in Patients with Manifest Autoimmunity: Observational Study," *Autoimmunity Reviews* 17, no. 11 (2018): 1078–80.

4. T. C. Wallace et al., "Dairy Intake Is Not Associated with Improvements in Bone Mineral Density or Risk of Fractures Across the Menopause Transition: Data from the Study of Women's Health Across the Nation," *Menopause* 27, no. 8 (2020): 879–86.

5. A. Trichopoulou et al., "Healthy Traditional Mediterranean Diet: An Expression of Culture, History, and Lifestyle." *Nutrition Reviews* 55, no. 11 (1997): 383–89; S. Dernini, "The Erosion and the Renaissance of the Mediterranean Diet: A sustainable Cultural Resource," *Quaderns de la Mediterrania* 16 (2011): 75–82; T. I. Gonzàlez, "The Mediterranean Diet: Consumption, Cuisine, and Food Habits," in *MediTERRA 2012: The Mediterranean Diet for Sustainable Regional Development,* ed. F. Mombiela (Paris: CIHEAM Sciences/Presses de Sciences Po, 2012), 115–32; N. R. Sahyoun et al., *Historical Origins of the Mediterranean Diet, Regional Dietary Profiles, and the Development of the Dietary Guidelines* (Totowa, NJ: Humana Press, 2016), 43–56; C. M. Lăcătuşu et al., "The Mediterranean Diet: From an Environment-Driven Food Culture to an Emerging Medical Prescription," *International Journal of Environmental Research and Public Health* 16, no. 6 (2019): 942.

6. M. De Lorgeril et al., "Mediterranean Alpha-Linolenic Acid–Rich Diet in Secondary Prevention of Coronary Heart Disease," *The Lancet* 343, no. 8911 (1994): 1454–59; M. De Lorgeril et al., "Mediterranean Diet, Traditional Risk Factors, and the Rate of Cardiovascular Complications After Myocardial Infarction: Final Report of the Lyon Diet Heart Study," *Circulation* 99, no. 6 (1999): 779–85; R. Estruch et al., "Retraction and Republication: Primary Prevention of Cardiovascular Disease with a Mediterranean Diet," *New England Journal of Medicine* 368 (2013): 1279–90; M. Sotos-Prieto et al., "Assessing Validity of Self-Reported Dietary Intake Within a Mediterranean Diet Cluster Randomized Controlled Trial among US Firefighters," *Nutrients* 11, no. 9 (2019): 2250.

7. J. Salas-Salvado et al., "Effect of a Mediterranean Diet Supplemented with Nuts on Metabolic Syndrome Status: One-Year Results of the PREDIMED Randomized Trial," *Archives of Internal Medicine* 168, no. 22 (2008): 2449–58; M. T. Mitjavila et al., "The Mediterranean Diet Improves the Systemic Lipid and DNA Oxidative Damage in Metabolic Syndrome Individuals: A Randomized, Controlled Trial," *Clinical Nutrition* 32, no. 2 (2013): 172–78; N. Di Daniele et al., "Impact of Mediterranean Diet on Metabolic Syndrome, Cancer, and Longevity," *Oncotarget* 8, no. 5 (2017): 8947–79; M. Finicelli et al., "Metabolic Syndrome, Mediterranean Diet, and Polyphenols: Evidence and Perspectives," *Journal of Cell Physiology* 234, no. 5 (2019): 5807–26.

8. O. Ajala et al., "Systematic Review and Meta-Analysis of Different Dietary Approaches to the Management of Type 2 Diabetes," *American Journal of Clinical Nutrition* 97, no. 3 (2013): 505–16; J. Salas-Salvadó et al., "Prevention of Diabetes with Mediterranean Diets: A Subgroup Analysis of a Randomized Trial," *Annals of Internal Medicine* 160, no. 1 (2014): 1–10; published correction appears in 169, no. 4 (2018): 271–272.

9. Shai et al., "Weight Loss with a Low-Carbohydrate"; F. M. Sacks et al., "Comparison of Weight-Loss Diets with Different Compositions of Fat, Protein, and Carbohydrates." *New England Journal of Medicine* 360, no. 9 (2009): 859–73; C. Haro et al., "Two Healthy Diets Modulate Gut Microbial Community Improving Insulin Sensitivity in a Human Obese Population," *Journal of Clinical Endocrinology Metabolism* 101, no. 1 (2016): 233–42.

10. N. Di Daniele et al., "Impact of Mediterranean Diet on Metabolic Syndrome, Cancer, and Longevity," *Oncotarget* 8, no. 5 (2017): 8947–79.

11. E. Toledo et al., "Mediterranean Diet and Invasive Breast Cancer Risk Among Women at High Cardiovascular Risk in the PREDIMED Trial: A Randomized Clinical Trial," *JAMA Internal Medicine* 175, no. 11 (2015): 1752–60.

12. E. H. Martínez-Lapiscina et al., "Mediterranean Diet Improves Cognition: The PREDIMED-NAVARRA Randomised Trial," *Journal of Neurology and l Neurosurgery Psychiatry* 84, no. 12 (2013): 1318–25; A. Knight et al., "A Randomised Controlled Intervention Trial Evaluating the Efficacy of a Mediterranean Dietary Pattern on Cognitive Function and Psychological Wellbeing in Healthy Older Adults: The MedLey Study," *BMC Geriatrics* (2015): 15:55; C. Valls-Pedret et al., "Mediterranean Diet and Age-Related Cognitive Decline: A Randomized Clinical Trial," *JAMA Internal Medicine* 175, no. 7 (2015): 1094–103.

13. J. E. de la Rubia Ortí et al., "Improvement of Main Cognitive Functions in Patients with Alzheimer's Disease After Treatment with Coconut Oil Enriched Mediterranean Diet: A Pilot Study," *Journal of Alzheimer's Disease* 65, no. 2 (2018): 577–87.

14. S. I. Katz et al., "Randomized-Controlled Trial of a Modified Mediterranean Dietary Program for Multiple Sclerosis: A Pilot Study," *Multiple Sclerosis Related Disorders* 36 (2019): 101403.

15. O. Ajala et al., "Systematic Review and Meta-Analysis."

16. J. L. Steiner et al., "Impact of Alcohol on Glycemic Control and Insulin Action," *Biomolecules* 5, no. 4 (2015): 2223–46; M. B. Esser et al., "Peer Reviewed: Prevalence of Alcohol Dependence Among US Adult Drinkers, 2009–2011," *Preventing Chronic Disease* 11 (2014); R. W. Wilsnack et al., "Gender Differences in Binge Drinking: Prevalence, Predictors, and Consequences," *Alcohol Research: Current Reviews* 39, no. 1 (2018): 57–76.

17. K. Bogusz et al., "Prevalence of Alcohol Use Disorder Among Individuals Who Binge Eat: A Systematic Review and Meta-Analysis," *Addiction* (2020). doi: 10.1111/add.15155.

# INDEX

# ABOUT THE AUTHOR

Sara Gottfried, MD, is a board-certified physician who graduated from Harvard Medical School and the Massachusetts Institute of Technology, and completed residency at the University of California at San Francisco. Over the past two decades, Dr. Gottfried has seen more than 25,000 patients, and specializes in identifying the root causes underlying her patients' conditions to achieve true and lasting health transformations, not just symptom management. To promote unprecedented health, she is likely to test her patient's DNA and next-generation biomarkers, and then prescribe a personalized lifestyle protocol, using primarily food (not drugs) plus other proven interventions to optimize the gene-environment interface. For each patient, she designs an N-of-1 trial to provide rapid information on whether the personalized prevention plan will improve outcomes. It's not "one method fits all." It's not disease-centered. It's not "fix 'em up and send 'em home." It's a mission to transform health care, one patient at a time.

Dr. Gottfried is a global keynote speaker who practices evidence-based integrative, precision, and functional medicine. She is a clinical assistant professor in the Department of Integrative Medicine and Nutritional Sciences at Sidney Kimmel Medical College, Thomas Jefferson University, and director of precision medicine at the Marcus Institute of Integrative Health. She has published three *New York Times*–bestselling books: *The Hormone Cure, The Hormone Reset Diet,* and *Younger.* Learn more at http://SaraGottfriedMD.com.